Profound Healing

Profound Healing

The Power of Acceptance
on the Path to Wellness

CHERYL CANFIELD

Healing Arts Press
Rochester, Vermont

Healing Arts Press
One Park Street
Rochester, Vermont 05767
www.InnerTraditions.com

Healing Arts Press is a division of Inner Traditions International

Note to the reader: This book is intended as an informational guide.
The remedies, approaches, and techniques described herein are meant
to supplement, and not to be a substitute for, professional medical care or
treatment. They should not be used to treat a serious ailment without
prior consultation with a qualified health care professional.

Library of Congress Cataloging-in-Publication Data
Canfield, Cheryl, 1947-
Profound healing : the power of acceptance on the path to wellness /
Cheryl Canfield ; foreword by Joseph Chilton Pearce.
p. cm.
Includes bibliographical references.
ISBN 0-89281-097-1 (pbk.)
1. Canfield, Cheryl, 1947—-Health. 2. Cervix
uteri—Cancer—Patients—United States—Biography. 3. Healing. I.
Title.

RC280.U8C365 2003
362.1'9699466'0092—dc21

2002154849

Printed and bound in the United States at Lake Book Manufacturing, Inc.

10 9 8 7 6 5 4 3 2 1

Text design and layout by Virginia Scott Bowman and Rachel Goldenberg
This book was typeset in Janson Text

Dedication

This book is dedicated to God and to peace and to the preservation of our beautiful planet;

to the guardians, guides, and friends from the heavenly realm who lovingly remind us of our spiritual roots and potential;

to my daughter, Cindy, who shares my laughter and my tears and who continues to teach me;

and to my friend Randal whose enthusiasm and encouragement supported me throughout the writing of this book.

Contents

Part Three: Reengaging Life

Part Four: Twelve Steps in the Healing Process

Foreword

So many books on healing flood the market today—making audacious claims, often opportunistic and self-serving—that I can seldom read one through. I have read this work of Cheryl Canfield's four times, however, and shall no doubt read it again. I carried the manuscript around with me for the first few weeks, rather as a warm companion, and still dip into it some two years later.

Canfield builds her book around several themes. First, she offers a play-by-play account of her experience with cancer—from the initial death sentence, to her eventual deliverance from that shadow—which she achieves without fanfare, and entirely on her own. Canfield shows us that a first step in healing is assuming responsibility for every aspect of our life, including learning all we can of the affliction facing us, and, as the Sufis say, "keeping the devil in front of us, in clear sight."

Second, she uses brief biographical glimpses into her background, not from the ego posturing of one who has held the grim reaper at bay single-handedly, but rather as a foundation on which her new understanding of cancer, disease in general, and health itself could take shape and be shared. Thus, Canfield's story proves far more than just an account of moving beyond illness. It is a story of transcendence and moving into new life.

Third, while subtly sensational in substance, the way of healing she describes is marked by quiet humility and understatement, from which a fresh insight into the human spirit unfolds. In claiming so little for herself, she offers so much to us all. The glimpses into her spiritual background are richly revealing, particularly her long association with that elusive giant of the spirit, Peace Pilgrim.

Throughout this book I found Canfield's modesty, integrity, and honesty so compelling that I flew to the West Coast to meet her. That personal contact was even more rewarding than the intellectual contact I experienced through her book—one of those rare occasions when one finds the author in person even more genuine and impressive than that person in print. She doesn't just walk her talk; she *is* her talk—so much so that her inner radiance is infectious and we carry something of it away with us.

Above all, Canfield shows that the onset of a disease, even a deadly one, can be the opening of an adventure of the spirit; the discovery of a wholly different aspect of life; and a challenge that can be every bit as life changing as life threatening. I have heard others speak of affliction as opportunity, but Canfield clearly demonstrates that disease and impending death can be a source of grace and liberation rather than a curse. This good news runs as a clear stream throughout her narrative. And here is a priceless hidden pearl in this work: at some point, in following her precepts for transcendence through forgiveness and nonjudgment, body healing becomes almost secondary to the many other levels of freedom and new life that open.

Surely readers will find their own gems in this work. More important, they may also find the incentive to undertake the simple journey into wholeness the book offers. Whether one is in boundless health, as was Peace Pilgrim, or facing crisis, as Cheryl was, the rewards will inevitably be great.

Joseph Chilton Pearce
Faber, Virginia
March, 2002

Acknowledgments

My gratitude goes to the many people who encouraged me and gave support throughout the writing of this book, as well as to all those whose inspiring stories are included herein.

I am most grateful to Joseph Pearce for his endorsement of my work and his support in getting this book to publication; for his introduction to Inner Traditions • Bear & Company; and for the foreword that he so generously contributed.

I deeply appreciate the support of my agent, Barbara Neighbors Deal, her belief in this project, and her valuable suggestions along the way.

The staff at Inner Traditions • Bear & Company have my heartfelt thanks for their professionalism and the care and support they demonstrated in all aspects of editing and production.

My gratitude flows abundantly to many friends, and particularly to Randal Churchill, whose steadfast enthusiasm and counsel kept me going through many difficult moments during the completion of this work.

Most of all I would like to thank my family—especially my parents, who have given me unconditional love and support; my daughter, Cindy; my son-in-law, Randy; and my grandsons, Matthew, Zachary, and Nathan, who bring immeasurable meaning to my life.

I thank the wonderful network of support in the little community of Groveland. I am fortunate to live amid abundant beauty in the foothills of Yosemite, with the delightful companionship of many friends (both two-footed and four-footed). Thanks especially to Bill Zachman, neighbor, friend, and computer consultant who came to my aid whenever I needed his invaluable assistance.

Finally, I would be remiss if I didn't mention the soulful presence of my cats during the process of writing. Socrates and Maxi have the ability to inspire me, console me, and make me laugh no matter how difficult the challenges before me.

Introduction

Mobilizing Our Inner Resources

Profound Healing was born out of my own experience with advanced cancer. What happens when we find out that the life we have taken for granted may soon end? What do we do with the flood of questions and emotions that pour in? "How can this be happening to me?" we ask in disbelief. "Why?"

What I discovered is that profound healing, healing from the inside out, is a do-it-yourself job. It is much more than a quick fix or the completion of some treatment or the cessation of a physical condition or disease. It requires the courage to look honestly and clearly at ourselves from the inside. It is about a willingness to face our deepest fears, look death itself in the face, and delve deep enough to find our unique purpose in this life.

How we react to any experience is a choice. "This is what life has offered me. What do I choose to do with it?" Until we are confronted by a life-threatening condition or major challenge, we can only imagine how we might act or feel. My first surprise was that this could happen to me. Here I was, teaching people to live healthy, fulfilling lives. What was I going to do now?

And then I realized that the choice was in my hands. I was a teacher, and it was time to get busy on my next assignment—learning and teaching how to die well. When I was able to accept this new reality, I was surprised to find a very strong sense of inner guidance

1

that kept surfacing and directing me through a journey I had never dreamed I would take.

My first steps were tentative, but my confidence grew as I became emboldened by an expanding inner reality. If my experience has taught me anything, it is that death is not to be feared. Life, as we experience its physical limitations, is always terminal. If death is a tragedy, it is only so to the degree to which we failed to live while on Earth.

Profound Healing takes into perspective the bigger picture of ourselves as spirit, separate from and much greater than the body. Of course it is our responsibility to take good care of our bodies at all times, and this is especially so in the event of a serious illness or catastrophic life event. Without the body we wouldn't be here to discover the opportunities and potential for profound growth and healing that are inherent in times of great challenge. This in itself is a major insight in reframing our perspective of illness and hardship: in facing difficult times we can expand our awareness to uncover an incredible array of inner resources that we might otherwise never have found.

While it is true that the recommended treatment for my advanced condition was so radical that I chose not to undergo medical intervention, this book is not a treatise to ignore the incredible advances in modern medical technology that exist to assist us. The disease process in my body was simply so advanced that I felt I wouldn't make it through the complex surgery; I chose instead to attempt to build up my immune system and sustain my body long enough to bring a few things to completion and make peace with my existence. Yet instead of coming to the end of the journey, I found the road stretched out before me.

People often ask me, "So what do you think it was that made you well?" There were so many steps along the way. Who can say at what point the body heals? I don't know. The ego likes to assert that healing has occurred, but a spiritual perspective is one of surrender. I never knew what the physical outcome would be or how much time I would have left. In retrospect, I did identify a series of steps in my personal journey that are included in this text. The steps can help open the channels of communication to the deeper parts of ourselves that spark our unique creativity and expression and lead to profound healing.

Illness can be seen as something to get rid of or as something to learn from. I chose to find out what I could learn. I know now that profound healing is not about surviving physical illness. It is about the limitlessness of spirit, and the freedom that comes from discovering that spiritual reality within. With that freedom, the experience of life enlarges a hundredfold, and it is possible to move from the microcosm of awareness into the macrocosm. It is not clinging to life that is important. It is what we do with life. While I see more clearly the underlying beauty and grandeur in all aspects of life, I also see the warning signs of greed and violence and immaturity that threaten to overtake the collective health and longevity of our species and our planet. We are all receiving a wake-up call, a call to personal responsibility, integrity, and compassion. These are the things that heal us. When enough of us have done sufficient inner healing and have matured to a certain level, we will begin to effect the external healing of our institutions and our world. Every thought we think, every action we take, influences the whole. When we do nothing we become part of the undoing. When we do something—even take one little step— we begin to heal ourselves and become part of healing the whole.

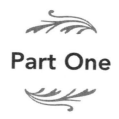

Part One

Preparing
for the Possibilities

1

Face to Face
with Mortality

Wealth and power pass like a dream,
beauty fades like a flower,
long life is gone like a wave.
WILLIAM BUCK

At the age of forty-one I was diagnosed with advanced cancer and told I might not live long enough to see the child in my daughter's womb. The news was incomprehensible.

I found my thoughts turning back to all the years leading up to that point in my life. There were so many things I still wanted to do. I wanted to know this baby that was going to be born. I wanted all of my grandchildren to know me. I had so many stories to tell. Would I have time to tell them? And I was still struggling to make sense of my many experiences. *Please, God,* I prayed, *let me live long enough to tie up my loose ends and complete the things I came into this life to do.*

It felt strange to ponder death as it loomed imminently near, and even more so because the face that looked back from the mirror wasn't yet fully weathered. I had held a rather romantic idea of death as a time when I would feel I had completed life's lessons. I would be old, certainly wiser than I currently felt, and ready to move on to that radiant place I had visited briefly during a near-death experience. But here I was, and I wasn't ready. There was still so much to learn and to do. I wanted to feel a sense of peace and completeness before I left this life. And I didn't want to be afraid.

The signs of illness had been a long time coming. Tiredness had plagued me for months, and at times a sharp pain in my abdomen caused me to double over. The first time it happened I was standing in the kitchen, and the pain brought me to my knees. Andy and I had been in the middle of an argument. *It's just emotional,* I told myself— until a routine pap smear showed abnormal cells.

I was reluctant to undergo the recommended colposcopy, a procedure which would entail snipping tissue samples from the cervix for biopsy. I tried to build up my immune system first, hoping to get my body back to normal before the test. I arranged to have some acupuncture treatments, enrolled in a class called Conscious Living, and paid even more attention to eating well and getting plenty of rest and exercise. I pulled out my old journals and started writing again. Writing tapped me into a greater awareness of my emotions, which I suspected I had been avoiding.

When I felt ready I made an appointment for the colposcopy. Cells taken from my cervix came back positive. I had cervical cancer. Moreover, the doctor found a lump in my breast.

It didn't seem possible. I wasn't a likely candidate for cancer. I practiced hatha yoga daily, followed a balanced vegetarian diet, and meditated. I led a retreat center and taught steps toward inner peace. I was teaching other people how to live healthy, balanced lives! Cancer didn't happen to people like me! This brought up a very uncomfortable feeling—humiliation. How could I be teaching others when I was so out of balance myself? Was I a hypocrite or an impostor? What was I doing wrong?

Dr. Turner wanted to do an immediate needle aspiration of the lump in my breast and a cone biopsy of the cervix. I wanted more time to build up my immune system. I knew my body was overloaded with years of emotional stress and loss.

Several weeks later I was walking down a hallway when I caught a glimpse of myself in a mirror at the end of the corridor. My skin appeared pale and transparent, like that of a disembodied apparition. The image sent a shiver up my spine. I made the call to schedule the cone biopsy.

I was on the table in the operating room, drowsy from the drug that had been given me and shaking from the cool temperature when Dr. Turner came in. "Get a blanket on her right now!" she demanded of a nearby nurse. She placed her hand on my leg and looked into my eyes with reassuring compassion. It was the last thing I remembered before succumbing to unconsciousness.

The silent peacefulness was broken by an unfamiliar nurse telling me to get my clothes on. That was odd. Where was I? Why weren't my clothes on? Then Andy was there, assisting the nurse as they tugged and pushed me into my clothes. I had arranged for Andy, now my ex-husband, to drive me home. He picked me up, literally, and carried me to the car.

I lay in the back seat where I closed my eyes and tried to still the sickening sensations in my stomach. Every lurch of the car during the hour's drive upset my stomach and head. Then I was back at Andy's house. My house. The house we had built with our own hands, only it wasn't mine anymore. Now I was a guest here. He carried me through the living room into a small bedroom.

My parents were staying in the other guest room while they waited for their new house to be ready. My brother Tim, his wife, Veronica, and their kids were living in a trailer on the property. We were a strange mixture of the Waltons and Murphy Brown. The idea struck me as funny, but the feeling turned into nausea.

It felt good to lie still, but the nausea and disorientation kept rising to the surface. Karen, my niece, stuck her head through the doorway, her little girl face lit up in smiles. I wanted to say something but I could only curl up tighter. I hoped to never feel this miserable again.

Five days later, on Easter Sunday, we were joined by Cindy and

Randy, my daughter and son-in-law, and their two sons. Cindy, pregnant with their third child, was feeling very sick. All of her pregnancies were difficult, and this one was following close on the heels of her last, before she'd even had a chance to recover her strength. Zachary was only a few months old. Cindy had been severely nauseated all day and stayed overnight with me to rest, while Randy took the kids home with him.

By morning Cindy was completely dehydrated, and I took her to the hospital and checked her in. In the afternoon I drove to my appointment with Dr. Turner. Her office had called on Good Friday to tell me that the lump in my breast had been benign and the results of my cone biopsy would be in after Easter.

I strode confidently toward the doctor's office. Mothering Cindy had bolstered my energy and strength. "Say, you're looking great!" Dr. Turner said warmly when she spotted me coming down the hallway.

"Thanks!" I responded, interpreting her comment to mean that all was well. "I feel pretty good, too, considering I've just come from admitting my daughter into the hospital." I felt so optimistic that I hadn't waited for an invitation to go on. "As soon as you give me the OK I'm going to pick up my two grandchildren so Cindy can rest when she gets home."

By then we had entered her office, and I flashed her a smile as I eased into a chair. My smile froze when I saw the muscles in Dr. Turner's face sag. "Oh-oh!" I said. "It looks like the news might not be so good." An alarm was going off in my stomach.

"I didn't want to spoil your Easter," she said. "The cancer is invasive. I'm so sorry. I took the largest cone section I've ever taken out of anybody, hoping to get it all."

Time and sound and distance all snapped out of sync. I tried to focus on Dr. Turner's words when she went over the lab tests, but the sounds floated around. I caught a word here and there, but they weren't coming together right. She talked about options. She said she hoped I wouldn't mind that she had already made an appointment for me with a gynecological oncologist. "This is something you just can't sit on," she finished. "You might not be here to see the child your daughter is carrying."

She showed me out a back door so I wouldn't have to go through the waiting room. As I started to leave she called, "Wait!" When I turned she wrapped her arms around me for a moment. I was physically and emotionally numb, but in some far away place I appreciated this gesture. Like an automaton I continued on to my car, got in, and started to drive. Before I reached the highway I was overcome by emotions and pulled over. Tears let loose. I was on my way to comfort Cindy, who was waiting, weak and vulnerable, in the hospital. How could I tell her, when she needed me so much, that I might not be here for long?

Two days later I was in Dr. Kinton's office. Still raw from the surgery, I found the examination excruciating. While I lay open-legged and vulnerable on the examining table, the doctor began describing in detail the radical surgery he believed was necessary. When he finished he drew a picture of my cervix to illustrate how the cancer had already traveled beyond the section of cervix that had been removed and was likely to have traveled outside of the uterus as well. This meant that even a radical hysterectomy would not be enough.

What Dr. Kinton proposed was something so delicate that not more than three hundred doctors in the country were trained to perform the operation. Surgery would entail removing not only my uterus but also an outer lying margin that was filled with nerves and muscles. Very delicate tubes would need to be lifted out, stripped back meticulously, and pulled out of the way of cutting. There would be inevitable damage, the doctor explained. Lymph nodes must go, fallopian tubes, uterus, cervix, and most of the vagina. Because the uterus lies against the bladder and rectum, it was possible that those areas could be damaged. The worst-case scenario would include the removal of my colon and the insertion of a bag on the outside of my body to collect waste. It was likely that I would not be able to urinate on my own following surgery and would need a permanent catheter.

With such delicate surgery it was inevitable that repair surgeries would be needed following the initial procedure. All of these things increased the potential of my developing heart problems. In addition, I knew that when lymph nodes in the groin area are removed, swelling and infections in the legs can be very serious. I'd read about a woman who'd had to have first one leg and then the other amputated after such a procedure. I don't know at what point the images that were forming in my mind began to show on my face, but the doctor glanced up as he finished and said, "You look overwhelmed."

"I don't think I want to live in the body that would be left," I blurted out. "I'm not afraid to die."

I left unspoken the thought that had popped into my awareness like a red neon light: if I had the surgery I would die on the operating table. Without the surgery I knew I might die, but I also knew it wasn't inevitable. No one can predict death. Life is both fragile and tenacious. I opted to trust my intuition.

The doctor was visibly upset when I told him I didn't want the surgery. "What are you going to do?" he asked.

"Research," I answered.

"But I've got all the books and research," he responded. "I'll send you the information to go over for yourself."

I thanked him sincerely and left. By the time I reached my car I had decided I would go to Mexico. I had been researching alternative cancer clinics in Tijuana for an article I was writing. How ironic that I would get a diagnosis of cancer during that process.

2

Weighing the Alternatives

Whatever you do, if you do it sincerely, will eventually become a bridge to your wholeness, a good ship that carries you through the darkness.

CARL JUNG

On Friday I drove to the Tijuana border. It was only days after my diagnosis and the reality hadn't fully sunk in. I was so preoccupied with the adventure of researching clinics that I was more tuned in to going after a good story than dealing with something as personally threatening as advanced cancer.

Cancer clinics are a lesser known side of Tijuana. The city's proximity to the U.S. border provides the geographic opportunity to offer treatments that are not recognized or accepted in the United States: Laetrile, enzymes, phytochemicals, chelation, cellular and electromagnetic processes—the list goes on. I drove into the International Motor Inn at the San Ysidro border crossing in the afternoon, just in time to catch the van that made daily rounds to some of the clinics in Mexico. It was the last run of the day, and though I wouldn't have a lot of time I'd be able to gather information and collect brochures.

American Biologies was the first stop. On the steps, looking oddly out of place, stood a couple in formal Amish attire. We exchanged greetings as I went inside for brochures. When I returned to the van I slid into a seat behind that couple, as yet the only passengers.

After quick introductions we began to exchange our stories. The woman had come for treatment of stomach cancer, accompanied by her husband. He had also been examined, and nose polyps were discovered. He looked drawn and tired from surgery done that day, and was leaning back with his eyes closed. A huge bandage covered his swollen nose.

"What kind of treatment are you receiving?" I asked the woman.

"Chemotherapy," she related, much to my surprise, "along with Laetrile." She went on to explain that the clinics were now taking advantage of conventional methods in conjunction with alternative therapies. "We're both very pleased with our treatments," she added.

The conversation drifted for a moment to their home in Pennsylvania and their livelihood of farming. Practices had changed dramatically over the years, and they now relied heavily on chemicals. I wondered to myself about the possible relationship between their cancers and the chemicals they used. "It seems you need to change with the times," the woman was saying. Startled by her comment, I inadvertently scanned her traditional costume, and we both laughed as she caught my glance.

The van was filling up with patients from other clinics. The last stop of the day was the Contreres Hospital, and the van was full when I returned. I squeezed myself into the back, my arms filled with brochures. Everyone seemed friendly, curious about one another and anxious to tell their stories. There were patients from Canada, England, Germany, and Australia, as well as the United States. Some were here for the first time; others were returning for checkups. Several talked about being cancer-free, or knowing others who were living cancer-free after treatment at one of the clinics.

It had been an exciting start. Back at the inn I spread out the brochures to acquaint myself with the available programs. Most included chemotherapy, radiation, or surgery as options to be used along with some combination of Laetrile, chelation, nutrition programs, live cell therapy, and others. I didn't feel drawn to any particular program. Live cell therapy was especially unappealing to me: I didn't eat animals and wasn't comfortable with the idea of having live cells from young calves injected into my body.

I started to feel queasy. What if I didn't find what I was looking for? Remembering a video I had seen about a facility called the Bio-Medical Center, I searched through the phone book and found the number. I called to make an appointment for an evaluation on Monday.

Saturday morning dawned on clear blue skies. It was tempting to enjoy a lazy day around the pool and sauna, but I wanted to visit more clinics before Monday. The only way I could do that was to drive across the border myself. I was apprehensive about the foreign laws and road signs but relaxed when I got out of crowded Tijuana and onto the main highway. With map in hand it was pretty much like driving along an unfamiliar road at home.

At Rosarita Beach I visited Dr. Donsbach's hospital. I enjoyed exploring the quaint little town, but every step was an effort. At this point the most moderate exercise caused my body to tremble.

On my way back I took a wrong turnoff, but divine Providence was with me. Right in front of me was the Manner Clinic, where a friend of mine had stayed for treatment of breast cancer. I had been impressed that she'd been allowed to keep her little dog with her in a private room. My knock on the door was met by a friendly gray-haired woman, who fondly remembered my friend and took me on a tour. I was even able to purchase a several months' supply of Laetrile, which I'd been looking for. My last stop before returning to the inn was the Gerson Clinic. The next day was definitely a time to rest and soak up the sun.

On Monday morning I woke up early, anxious to get to the Bio-Medical Center for my evaluation. The van was full, and upon arrival we all joined a line that was already gathering in front of the reception area. After filling out a registration form, I was directed down a hall where I was greeted by a smiling man in a white lab coat. He handed me a cup for a urine sample, and when I returned with it I was given a paper with the same number that had been on my cup.

I was also handed a blue gown and sent to a waiting area that was lined with dressing rooms along one side.

There were several people sitting and standing in blue robes when I emerged from the dressing room. The one-size-fits-all gowns had loose, draping arms, so that with a little imagination we looked like a gathering of blue angels. There were nervous giggles as more and more people stepped out of the dressing rooms, and a spontaneous camaraderie arose among us. Old-timers (those who had been here before) started telling their stories, and soon everyone was swapping experiences.

The room was full when the same smiling man in the white lab coat entered. "Here comes the vampire for our blood!" joked someone. The technician picked up the first vial and called out my number. Everyone gathered around to support and cheer me as deep-red blood was drawn from my arm into the clear tube.

From there I was sent to the X-ray lab where films were taken of my abdomen, chest, and back. After that I got back into my clothes and went to the lobby to wait.

The lobby was a big, comfortable room outside of which a veranda overlooked the city. I wandered out and found a man leaning on a railing in the corner, smoking a cigarette. When he turned around he looked like one of the saddest people I'd ever seen. We spoke, and he told me that two weeks earlier, feeling perfectly fine, he had gone in for a routine exam. Xrays showed he had advanced lung cancer. His doctor said it was too late to do anything and told him to go home and put his affairs in order. He had flown to the clinic from Minnesota looking for a miracle cure, but he couldn't give up the thing that was killing him. He stomped out his cigarette as we talked.

When my number was called I was led into an office upstairs. The doctor, a slight, dark-haired woman, asked about my condition and history before ushering me onto an examining table. I was given a complete exam and then sent back to the lobby to wait while she consulted with the other doctors and came up with a treatment plan.

It was late afternoon when I got through the last line of the day. I was given a six-month supply of an herbal tonic, TST-25, vitamin C (which I was told to gradually build up to ten grams a day), calcium and iron pills, Pau D'Arco tea, an antibiotic for an infection that had shown up in one of my lab tests, Halox for use in my drinking water and as a douche, and a list of diet recommendations.

The van dropped me off at the inn. That was it. I had imagined that I would check into a clinic where doctors and nurses would monitor my treatments, as my friend had done. There would be a support staff to plan out and serve nutritious meals and fresh juices. I would rest my much fatigued body, soak up the sun on a white sandy beach, and visualize my immune system gobbling up cancer cells. Now here I was—alone—and I had to start working out my own plan. My energy waned. Tears marked the passing miles on the long drive home.

When I arrived a letter from Dr. Kinton was waiting for me, along with the information he had promised. He was alarmed by the position I was taking:

> I confess that I have never met anyone prior to yourself who felt that dying of cervical cancer would be preferable to the potential complications of treatment. Sending you this assortment of summaries of the operative complications is an extraordinarily one-sided view, as it does not take into account the prolonged misery associated with death from this kind of cancer. I feel that I'm qualified to address that issue because I have had the opportunity to care for a fair number of people who have not been curable when they met me.
>
> I can tell you from experience that this is neither a pretty nor an easy death. You told me that you are not afraid of dying and I see that as commendable and worthy of respect, however, there are a lot of different ways to die. While you may not wish to compromise your quality of life to postpone the inevitable you are currently being offered the chance to influence how you die. Death from cancer of the cervix is frequently a prolonged, extremely

painful, lingering, bleeding, and wasting sort of death. I am aware that you are concerned that you will bankrupt your parents in the process of being treated. Being cared for by them and having them watch this process and know you chose it may be more of a burden to them than any fiscal distress you could possibly inflict.

I don't know how you feel about doctors but I know that it is not uncommon amongst people of my generation to regard them as misguided and greedy at best. Something that didn't come up in our interview that bears mention is that I work on salary from the University. I have no financial interest whatsoever in whether you are treated or not. However, I have taken care of too many people dying of cervical cancer not to feel that the pain and immobility and bleeding and infection and odor from rotting tumor (while a "natural" event) is more of a compromise of your quality of life and that of those taking care of you than using a catheter after surgery or any of the other complications that you will see described at such length in the accompanying material.

Although I have no financial interest in your decision, I do feel, having met you, that I have a personal stake in convincing you not to put yourself and your loved ones through your dying of cancer unnecessarily.

His description of death by cancer and certainty in his position fanned the flames of my fear. I was well aware of how powerful our minds are in manifesting whatever we take in as a belief. Already I felt alone and vulnerable. I knew that I could potentially die from this cancer. But I felt certain that I would die on the operating table. How could Dr. Kinton possibly understand? My intuition would seem so irrational to his scientific mind. I decided not to see him. Instead, I made an appointment with Dr. Turner.

I was very anxious as I sat in the waiting room. I knew she was expecting me to set a date for surgery, and here I was with my herbal tonic from Mexico. Inside her office, Dr. Turner listened as I told her about my trip. There was a brief silence when I finished. "Western medicine doesn't have the corner on healing," she said slowly. "I'm not going to abandon you." Then she asked if she could see my treatment plan from Mexico and make a copy of it. I was delighted to show her. She copied it immediately, handing me back the original. "I'm not following the plan entirely," I confided. "There are some things I'm not doing and others I'm adding."

I jumped as her hand slammed down on the desk in front of her. "Damn it, Cheryl!" she exclaimed. "You won't listen to anyone." I was embarrassed and could feel myself shaking, but I wanted her support, so I forced myself to continue. I pointed to the TST-25 on the sheet in front of her. "Isn't that testosterone?" I asked. "And if I'm not mistaken, isn't the idea of taking this male hormone meant to stop the production of estrogen? Estrogen feeds some types of cancer, but not cervical cancer, right? And there are several potential side effects. Is there any reason you know of that it might be useful for me?" She shook her head and I could feel my courage returning. "I also picked up a few months' supply of Laetrile and some enzymes. It probably can't hurt." She didn't say anything, but I thought I detected a smile.

3

Exploring Death

God allows us to experience the low points of life in order
to teach us lessons we could not learn in any other way.
The way to learn these lessons is not to deny the feelings
but to find the meanings underlying them.

STANLEY LINDQUIST

It wasn't death itself I was afraid of. It was all the things in Dr. Kinton's letter that frightened me. His words painted awful images of prolonged misery from a wasting, rotting illness. What if the process were to become overwhelming? What if my family suffered from my choices? What if I became so weak that I lost my bodily functions and had to be cleaned up after?

These thoughts were agonizing. I began to do research on how to take my own life. In my heart I knew that I couldn't escape whatever lessons life dealt, but I felt guilty even considering causing my family the kind of suffering the doctor had described. I felt like I had to know there was a way out if I ran out of resources.

I did my research quietly because I didn't want anyone to feel guilt or complicity if I decided to opt for such a choice. I also kept this research private because I felt ashamed—not just for having thoughts about taking my own life, but because I felt there was a stigma of failure attached to having cancer.

Since returning from Mexico I had moved with my little dog, Plato, into a U-shaped complex with a double row of studio apartments back to back. Each unit had a small bay window that looked out onto a grassy courtyard lined with rose bushes full of red and pink and yellow blossoms. It was charming despite its location on Main Street, surrounded by commercial businesses. The low-income residents were mostly transient and elderly.

Inside I set about to create a healing environment, surrounding myself with all the things that I loved. I hung favorite photos and nature scenes on the walls and started an inspiration file for poetry and uplifting stories. More often than not I would have some inspirational message taped to my bathroom mirror as a regular reminder. My small bookcase was filled with books on poetry, philosophy, spirituality and art, and I loved to have candles and fresh flowers around. I played my favorite music and watched videos on nature and healing. Plato kept me company and I loved to feel his warm body against my feet when I slept.

It was difficult to let go of the tempo and productivity I was used to. Now my days were filled with taking care of myself and preparing special foods and juices. The kitchen counter, covered with rows of vitamins and minerals and herbs, looked like a pharmacy. A list of supplements was taped on the wall with a schedule and instructions for taking the proper amounts of each supplement. I felt guilty that I was spending so much time on self-care and sleep. But I was tired. Many times a day I would find myself drifting off and sinking into oblivion.

While my weakened body needed rest, another part of me was awakening. My intuition was becoming especially keen. Sleep began to take on a new quality. It was like rolling out of one body into another as I drifted, not just between wakefulness and sleep, but between my dense physical body and a lighter etheric one.

Sleep became my other world, where I would meet with a group of people who were familiar to me in much the same way people I'm close to in my waking state are familiar. There was a natural affection among us, and we were further bonded by working together. Our various projects involved manipulating energy rather than physical things. On one occasion we used our combined energy to relieve pressure along a particularly volatile fault line in the Earth. We weren't able to prevent slippage, but we helped to lessen the severity. At other times we concentrated our prayers, holding individuals of power and influence in a circle of light.

During these periods my awareness seemed as clear as when I was awake, except that my body seemed very light, composed more of energy than matter. When it was time to wake up, that side would begin to dim and this side would become more clear. Sometimes in the middle I would be aware of both sides before rolling into this heavier body.

At other times during my sleep state, I found myself in a classroom. Sometimes the instruction came to a group I was part of, but the things I remembered most clearly were imparted when I was alone with a teacher.

The first time I'd had a lucid dream–like experience occurred just prior to the cancer diagnosis. While asleep and dreaming, I had become aware of a large outdoor amphitheater where I was sitting on one of the high benches looking down. In the center a figure was talking and making big gestures with his arms. The first few rows of seats were filled with people who were focused on the speaker. It looked like something important was going on, and I wanted to climb down and get close enough to hear, but I felt very tired and too heavy to move.

Then I became aware of an old man with a long white beard sitting next to me. His sparkling eyes, unlike the rest of him, didn't look old at all. He started talking to me about my health and noted that my body wasn't absorbing B vitamins very efficiently and that I could give more attention to balancing my diet. He talked for some time about specific B vitamins and how they affected energy. I was interested in how I had come to be in this condition. He said it wasn't really important to know, but it was the result of having consumed more than a little wine in a previous life. "You see," he explained, "even while in one body, you are affecting not only that body, but building the strengths and weaknesses of the next."

I was so excited to look up the information he was giving me that I woke up. I jumped up immediately and found my nutrition almanac. Sure enough, the text spelled out in detail what the old man had been describing to me.

The active nature of my sleep state, as I dealt with the cancer, relieved my feelings of guilt about sleeping so much. I trusted these deeper senses, and it felt good to go with the flow. My body was tired. It was comforting to know that, as I rested it, I was getting the benefit of learning and working on a different level. I came to love the in-between state just before I was completely awake. It was a tingly, euphoric place where I felt held in the balance between this physical life and the other—never knowing which it would ultimately be.

On an intellectual level I continued to struggle with the idea of suicide as a last resort. Then one night, in that altered state during sleep, I was reminded that every soul comes in with a life plan and that the moment of death cannot be altered without ramifications. Everything that happens serves some purpose even when it seems to make no sense. A bird struggles to break out of its shell or a butterfly to emerge from its cocoon. From the outside it looks like a painful struggle, but if we interfere with this natural process and try to hasten the transition, the baby bird will suffer or the butterfly will not fly. I began to see death in the same way. The process of dying, no matter how painful, would prepare me to fly. I woke up in the morning knowing that I would never again be tempted to hasten my departure from this body.

But what about pain? What if it became unbearable? This had been my fear. But it was the fear of pain, rather than pain itself, that was unbearable. Surrendering to pain, I was learning, can usher in an altered state that leads to liberation. Every precious moment contains an opportunity, and the greatest realization and transcendence may come at the time of transition. In that last instant the darkness may be pierced, or some lesson completed. If the time is cut short the lesson will be repeated at another time, until it is complete. That is the spiritual lesson: there are no shortcuts, only postponements.

I also feared that I would become a burden to the people I loved most. On the other hand, I did realize that if the situation were reversed I wouldn't hesitate to care for a loved one. Why would my loved ones not care for me with the same satisfaction that I would feel in their place? And if I could keep an attitude of appreciation and even humor, it would be that much easier for everyone. Somewhere inside I knew that we make such pacts before coming into this life, but fear had blurred my remembrance.

I was already learning how to die. It is as natural as being born, even if it comes with some struggle, as does birth. When the time is right we roll out of our bodies in the same easy way I was rolling out when I entered the other dimension during sleep. The only difference is that in death the cord that binds us to our bodies disconnects.

Upon waking I remembered the realizations that had come in my sleep. I felt the lifting of a tremendous burden. A great feeling of safety and comfort accompanied these new ideas. I knew I could handle whatever experiences came in the process of dying. I knew that I could help my loved ones to deal with my death by my own acceptance of my condition, whatever it might be. A powerful teaching had broken through the veil of forgetfulness. I felt wonderful. This might be my last challenge—to learn and to teach how to die well.

It would be wonderful if the deep insights gained in such moments stayed forever, but I found I would forget if I didn't make an effort to remember. Like so many people, I would get caught up in the busyness of life, of just making ends meet or meeting deadlines. Part of me was driven to compare myself to others. An inner critic was frequently available to keep me humble: "You're still trying to figure out where to go and everyone else is already there. Run, run, run—you'll never catch up!" said the voice that caused my stomach to knot and my insides to cringe. How ironic that a group of cells in my body had taken up the chant to run, run, run, and were reproducing out of control.

4

Buying Time

Time is a sort of river of passing events, and strong is its current; no sooner is a thing brought to sight than it is swept by and another takes its place, and this too will be swept away.

MARCUS AURELIUS

Time is that precious commodity in life that is so easily taken for granted. When I thought I might not have much left, I wanted only to do what I could to buy more. The most pressing need was to support my body and maintain my current health status while I worked on establishing a sense of inner peace and completion.

Nature has always been a model for me, and I trusted my body's natural process. If my body was producing a profusion of cancer cells, there must be a reason. Cause is a somewhat nebulous concept, encompassing many dimensions and complexities, but if I could only find some trigger I might be able to disarm the cancer. In the meantime I would continue to do research. We don't often know what we're working on at the time we're in the middle of it. It is in retrospect that we gain perspective. When I looked inside myself the advice that came was always the same: *Find out everything you can about cancer and then follow your intuition.*

I started by reading books on nutrition that related specifically to cancer and then I weighed what I read against my intuition. I used that inner guidance for everything—even when adding a new vitamin or herb to my regimen. I would retreat into a receptive state of meditation and wait for the subtle feeling that I thought of as my "no" sense or my "yes" sense. When it came I didn't question it. I knew from experience that questioning would only take it into the yo-yoing of rationalization, which so easily leads to confusion. I just accepted the feeling. Yes. No. I followed the intuition that came.

The best way to deal with something you're afraid of is to get acquainted with it, so I learned everything I could about cancer. One of the things I read is that cancer doesn't grow in oxygen. The particular type of cancer I had tends to metastasize to the lungs, so I reasoned that oxygenating my lungs would be a practical step toward preventing its spread.

I took up jogging. Every morning Plato and I would go out at sunup. At first I was so weak that I could barely jog half a block, but I built up my endurance until I could finish three miles. It was never effortless; it was hard work. But it felt good. It was an accomplishment I was proud of, and it helped me to feel stronger.

On the streets in the early morning, Plato and I made an assortment of acquaintances. First there were the dog walkers. Dogs are great for overriding privacy barriers. They barge right in with total disregard for personal boundaries. We made friends with many dogs and their owners.

We also discovered a small population of homeless people. We were living in a fairly small town with a population of fifty thousand, and the homeless weren't that visible during the height of the day. But in the early morning they could be found sleeping behind some tree in a vacant lot or awake and out on the streets in surprising number. At first the homeless individuals we passed wouldn't look at me or Plato. They walked by with eyes directed forward, usually giving us a wide berth or even crossing the street to avoid us.

I had read that many people who become homeless start to feel invisible because most of us look away from them, and that a large percentage of the homeless who start out with no mental illness often become psychologically disturbed in time. Homelessness comes with a great stigma. It wasn't difficult to imagine the pain behind some of the blank faces we passed.

The pace of my life had slowed down considerably; things that had once seemed incidental or vague now came more into focus. I felt connected to the people on the streets and started greeting the forlorn figures who passed by pushing shopping carts piled high with meager possessions. For a long time no one responded. Then one morning one of the regulars smiled down at the ground when I said hello. After that it was like a chain reaction as more and more of the blank faces we passed in the early morning dared to look out from behind the walls they had built. No one actually spoke, but I could feel the bonds growing between us as eyes began to meet mine with trust, and worn-out faces lit up with a smile. It was exhilarating to watch the formerly blank faces transformed by a simple greeting.

At home Plato was the darling of our very modest apartment complex. Animals weren't allowed, but I had pleaded my case with the landlord, explaining my situation to him, and he had agreed to a dog as long as I cleaned up after him and made sure he wasn't a nuisance to the neighbors. Far from being perceived as a nuisance, Plato was a magnet for people's affection. Helen, a schizophrenic woman, would shuffle by every day with a cup of coffee spilling out of one shaking hand and a prized morsel of food for Plato in the other. A steady procession of people made its way past my window each day, hoping to catch a glimpse of the little dog and calling out his praises when they spotted him. When the weather was good I left the door open with Plato on a leash so he could wiggle and squeak his pleasure when a member of his adoring audience came by.

On the opposite side of the courtyard my neighbor Bob would yell across whenever he saw us, calling out to me to bring Plato over. Whenever I did, Bob's pale blue eyes would water over, probably as much from the alcohol he constantly consumed as from his emotions, but he appeared genuinely pleased when Plato jumped onto his lap.

Bob whizzed around the sidewalks in his electric wheelchair, almost always inebriated and with a cigarette dangling from his lips. His body was emaciated and his sagging skin looked ancient. Bob was dying from lung cancer. He constantly complained about life and all the hard knocks he had received. He told me one day that his doctor had given him permission to smoke and drink all he wanted. "Indulge yourself. You haven't got anything to lose." Bob related the doctor's words as he choked from his chronic cough and took a swig of whiskey.

I looked at this sad old man who was destroying himself and realized how easy it would be to get pulled into his self-pity. Instead, I found myself saying, "You could stop smoking, Bob. And you could stop drinking. There are a lot of things you could do for yourself." His eyes opened wide in amazement, and I immediately regretted the words that had slipped out.

But after that day Bob sought me out relentlessly. He wanted to hear the truth, as painful as it was. Some deep part of him knew, as we all do, that it is never too late to take responsibility for the precious life we are given. From the bigger perspective, we take our state of consciousness and our addictions right over with us. Every action in the present creates the future, and we carry it with us like a seed from this life to the next.

Over the next few months Bob related bits of his life story to me. His biggest regret was that he had deserted his wife and alienated himself from his only child, a daughter who was living in Las Vegas. I encouraged him to contact her, and eventually he did. He was in tears telling me that she actually wanted to see him; she even offered to send him plane tickets to visit her. In an amazing act of will, Bob stopped drinking in order to make the trip. He didn't want his daughter to see him in his usual drunken state. He came back radiantly aglow and died shortly afterward. I know he had resolved one of the issues that had held him hostage—his regret over the loss of connection with his daughter. I hope he had also begun to resolve his feeling of powerlessness in dealing with the events of his life.

It was easy, I knew, to feel powerless in the face of things that feel out of our control. The more I read about cancer the more I realized that the prevailing attitude was to attempt to control and manipulate and overpower the condition, often treating it with overkill and destroying healthy cells along with the cancer. Rather than strengthening the body's natural process of healing, treatments routinely compromised patients' immune systems.

I was struck by the warlike terms and theories that were being applied to disease in general. Having turned our bodies into battlegrounds, we were doing battle with the enemy, the healthy tissues being sacrificed like the civilian casualties in a real war. Even the alternative approach of visualization used imaginary weapons to defeat of the enemy within, with massive armies employing high-tech weapons to destroy the bad guys.

I read statistics on the relative success of visualization and struggled to implement that technique, trying to imagine wiping out cancer cells. My attempts only left me feeling frustrated. This model just didn't fit for me. I didn't want to be at war with my body. I was a pacifist, an idealist who believed, from the deepest part of me, in the power of overcoming evil with good, and hatred with love.

Something important was missing, but I couldn't put my finger on it. I don't believe in random happenings. I do believe that from our limited perspective we don't usually see the whole picture. Simply cutting out the cancer cells, whether through surgery, visualization, or psychic healing, was ignoring an important message. What was cancer telling me?

Looking for clues I reviewed the different aspects of my life. I pulled out the five guidelines for a good life that my spiritual mentor had outlined. The first one was: A means of livelihood that is useful to society—something you enjoy doing. Admittedly my livelihood was currently limited, but I got a lot of fulfillment from the tasks I gave myself. Whenever a homeless person responded to my greeting or someone was drawn to my door, I would acknowledge these seemingly insignificant happenings as my particular assignment for the day.

The second guideline was: Inspirational things in your life—items that lift you up, such as special music or words or the beauty of nature. That was easy to work on. I loved filling my environment with inspiration and although my actual contact with nature was limited in the city, I loved the trees that lined the streets. I loved watching the sky in its multitude of faces and smelling the roses that bloomed outside my door. It was good to be reminded of the natural world.

The third guideline was: Good living habits—regular exercise, sunshine, and fresh air, food that nourishes the body, plenty of rest, and good thoughts. I was consciously including all of those things in my daily life, though I caught myself occasionally slipping on the last. "Junk thoughts can destroy you even more quickly than junk foods!" I could hear my mentor say.

The fourth guideline was, "A path of service—something you do with an outgoing motive to be of service, without thought of receiving anything in return." My living situation made fulfilling this one particularly easy. All around me were elderly people and variously challenged individuals who appeared at my door for a kind word or appreciation, and in turn they showered me with gifts in the form of food or flowers or small treasures. And if word got around that I wasn't up and about on a particular day, neighbors would come by, hobbling on artificial hips or leaning on canes to offer to bring me whatever I might need from the store. When I think of it, my most valuable service to them might have been allowing them to be of service to me.

Then there was the final guideline: "Time spent alone each day in meditation or receptive silence." When I lived in the country, my walking had been my time for meditation, but now there was activity all around when I walked. I realized I wasn't taking time to sit in silence. Why do people so often put off or forget what is easiest to take care of? I decided to pay more attention to creating quiet time.

As I relaxed into a quiet state of meditation one day, an image spontaneously came to mind of my cancer cells as young, unreasoning children. Bombarded by the stress that had overwhelmed me in recent years, they felt that their lives were being threatened. In panic they had begun reproducing rapidly in a frantic effort to survive, not realizing that this rapid reproduction was going to kill their host, my body, and ultimately themselves in the process.

I was profoundly struck by the image. I visualized going inside to gather up the cancer cells. I embraced them as I would young, frightened children, assuring them that they were no longer alone or helpless. They could stop reproducing. I was in charge now and I would take care of them. I felt an instant response as a feeling of peacefulness spread throughout my body. I didn't know if I would live or die, but I knew that on a spiritual level I had experienced a profound sense of healing.

5

Tying Up Loose Ends

Not to forgive is to be imprisoned by the past,
by old grievances that do not permit life
to proceed with new business.

ROBIN CASARJIAN

Life had become like a day that was about to end, and I didn't want to rest until the clutter had been picked up. I always feel more clear when things are organized, so I got out my journal and wrote down everything I could think of that I wanted to complete or do in whatever time remained. I was already following a treatment plan for my body. Now it was time to move into the more challenging areas of mind and spirit.

Keeping a positive mental attitude was at the top of the list. I outlined a plan to begin each day with a sense of appreciation. Every morning when I woke up I would keep my eyes closed for a while and pay attention to any lingering memories from my sleep state, going over any insights or dreams, and making a point to remember anything that might be significant enough to write down. Then I would direct my thoughts to gratitude and appreciation for the day before me.

Next I would mentally scan the inside of my body from head to toe, paying attention to any feelings and enjoying that tingly floating sensation that lingered briefly as I came into wakefulness. Most of the time I woke up feeling good, but on occasion I noticed jabbing pains in my lower abdomen. When that happened I would rest my hands there, feeling the warmth and visualizing the radiant energy of my palms penetrating and spreading throughout the area. I had gotten the idea after waking up several times in the middle of the night on my stomach, with the palms of my hands pressed underneath me against my abdomen. It wasn't a position I was accustomed to, but it somehow felt good.

When I was ready to open my eyes I would enter the world slowly, focusing on the things I loved as I looked around in the soft early light. Plato would be waiting patiently for my eyes to meet his, and then he would bounce up happily beside me, licking his appreciation all over my face and making me laugh. That marked the end of quiet reverie, but now I could pull out my journal to make notes while Plato pranced around in anticipation of the rest of our routine. We would open the blinds to look out onto the rose bushes, and then open the door so he could bound out to roll and frolic on the grass in the courtyard.

In my journal I wrote down my intention to bring the awareness of appreciation into the rest of my day. Writing things down reminded me to continue to move my inspirations into action. This one was fairly easy. The threat of losing something opens wide the door of appreciation. I was keenly aware of the preciousness of the smallest experiences—seeing puffy clouds against a blue sky, smelling fragrant roses, watching a smile break across the face of little Zachary, my youngest grandson, when he discovered something new. My heart easily overflowed with love.

But along with the cheerful and bright aspects of being alive, negative feelings were also coming up as I reviewed my history. Years earlier I had consciously embarked on a mystical path of awareness based on a faith that everything is divinely ordered. From this per-spective nothing happens randomly. On some level I understood that everything that had ever happened to me was for my own good. Every person and every event that had ever come into my life had come for a reason. In every situation, I believe, we are given oppor-tunities to learn and to teach; we give and receive. It was fruitless to try to understand with human logic why certain difficult things had happened. The only way to find permanent relief was to forgive, let go, and move on.

Knowing, however, is not the same as doing. I still felt the sting of lingering resentment and hurt. I also knew that those feelings were draining precious energy into the past so that I had less available to me in the present. I didn't like looking back, but if I wanted to be at peace I felt I had to sort it all out.

Forgiveness is an important principle I'd been teaching for years. There is no lasting healing without forgiveness, so if I really wanted to heal, I had to move beyond theory to practice. Being a victim of circumstances or people was incongruent with my spiritual perspective.

I made a list of everyone I could think of toward whom I held even slightly negative feelings, and started writing letters to them in my journal. After writing each letter I would read it as though I were the person receiving it, and then I would answer the letter as the other person. Very often being the other person not only broadened my perspective but actually changed it. At first I was consciously directing the communications, but after a while the characters (I and the other person) began to speak for themselves, and I became more of an observer. I wrote letters back and forth until both perspectives felt resolved or until there was a reciprocal agreement to let go and say goodbye.

The more I repeated this exercise the more I truly understood that every experience I'd ever had—especially interactions with others that continued to bother me—gave me an opportunity to learn. Every memory I reviewed offered an opportunity to test the strength of my beliefs. In any case, *it was only myself and my actions or reactions that I had ever been responsible for.*

I had already known this, but now I was absorbing the lesson more deeply. Forgiveness was really about taking responsibility for myself. I didn't have to accept or excuse any wrongdoing on the part of someone else; I only had to cut the bond of resentment that held me in bondage to that person.

My goal, more than ever, was to be able to respond from a loving and responsible place. As I wrote the "forgiveness letters" my focus shifted from how the other person had hurt me to what my actions or reactions had been. I asked myself what I might do differently now or what I might have done then to protect myself and stay centered and confident. I wrote until I could see from both my perspective and the other person's without judgment or guilt; at that point we were free to go our own ways without strings of resentment holding us back.

The process worked well until I got to a recent, more painful wound. Like it or not, the deep-seated negative feelings blotted out my best intentions. I could feel myself shrinking into a feeling of helplessness. I wanted to be strong and free to move on and heal, but I felt stuck. I turned to the Letters to God section of my journal and wrote: "Dear God, I want to forgive but I can't honestly let these feelings go. Since I don't know what else to do, I'm giving it to you. Please forgive this person in my name until I'm ready to do it myself."

As I wrote the words, I accepted that I sincerely wanted to forgive, and until that was possible I was leaving the burden in higher hands. My feelings of guilt and failure were dissolved in time. Later, when I looked back, I realized that the emotional triggers were gone. No memory brought up any sting or resentment. There was nothing left to forgive.

If we're willing to look deep enough, I discovered, we can see that no good comes from making another person the bad guy; blaming others only keeps us stuck in the role of victim. As long as my state of mind depended on another person to realize his or her mistake and repent, I was held in bondage. Yet I was the warden holding the key— and any time I wanted to, I could set myself free.

I couldn't be in charge of anyone else's attitudes and actions, but I always had control over my own. It was up to me to be discerning in my actions and reactions, doing what I needed to do to support and protect myself emotionally and physically, then leaving what I couldn't control in higher hands. Looking back, it was only when I had reacted in ways that were out of harmony with my spirit, or not taken action when I needed to, that I had lost my self-respect and felt beaten down.

The key to all of these exercises was honesty. To really heal, I knew I had to be completely honest with myself and find a way over each hump, one at a time. One of the most difficult challenges was coming to terms with the loss of a relationship that I had thought would be lifelong. I directed a lot of guilt and blame toward myself. There must be something wrong or unlovable about me. To prove this, I had even gone on and failed in a subsequent relationship.

Trying to figure out how to forgive myself was the most difficult test yet. What had I done wrong? I pondered over it and wrote about it. I squirmed and blanched and noted all my imperfections. I cried, I agonized, I yearned to be someone else. It was a long struggle.

Eventually I got to the other side. I realized that if I was truly going to be honest I couldn't look at my faults and mistakes without also looking at my other qualities. Ultimately, I reviewed the whole and found someone that I liked. There was no monster here. There was a sincere, sometimes confused person, someone willing to tough it out and make it right, someone who had a great compassion for life and learning and other people. I liked her; I liked myself.

Once I got to that point I was able to uncover years of buried resentment and anger toward the partner who had left me. I had taken all the responsibility onto myself as a way to protect him from any further hurt; I had made our problems all my fault. I turned again to my journal and wrote out my pain in a letter to him. I imagined being him and let him pour out his pain in a letter to me. In the end I was able to find the closure that had been so long coming in that relationship. I even found that I was able to love him in an impersonal way. I could respect that he was a separate individual dealing with his own lessons. Now I could reaffirm what I'd always known—that my wholeness and happiness come from within, not from circumstances or people outside of me. I live with a basic joyfulness about life simply because I choose to.

I appreciated the opportunity to be doing this work. It had come as a result of dealing with cancer, which I was also coming to appreciate in itself. Teachers come in many forms.

In my struggle to come to terms with forgiveness, I recalled a remarkable story I had once read about. It was from a book called *Return from Tomorrow* by George Ritchie. As a soldier in 1945, Ritchie was sent into Germany to give medical help to newly liberated prisoners. One of the concentration camp inmates had been given the nickname of Wild Bill because of his resemblance to the old Western hero. Wild Bill was working with the American soldiers because he knew several languages and was a good interpreter. At the end of long days the American soldiers would be tired and ready to quit, but Bill would press on. "We have time for this old fellow," he would say. "He's been waiting to see us all day."

Ritchie assumed that Wild Bill had only recently been incarcerated because, unlike the others, he had bright eyes, he stood tall and straight, and he wasn't emaciated. He was exceptional in many respects. Despite the fact that hatred among different nationalities in the camps ran almost as deep as hatred against the Germans, Wild Bill was loved by everyone. When Ritchie saw Wild Bill's papers he was amazed to find that he'd been there since 1939. "For six years he had lived on the same starvation diet, slept in the same airless and disease-ridden barracks as everyone else, but without the least physical or mental deterioration."

Feelings against Germans ran so strong in the camps that some of the liberated prisoners had already gone into nearby towns with guns to shoot Germans on sight. The Americans were working to try to prevent the shootings, and Wild Bill worked with them, talking to the different groups and enjoining them to practice forgiveness.

Talking with Wild Bill one day, Ritchie said, "It's not easy for some of them to forgive. So many of them have lost members of their families." Wild Bill then told his own story for the first time:

"We lived in the Jewish section of Warsaw—my wife, our two daughters and our three little boys. When the Germans reached our street they lined everyone against a wall and opened up with machine guns. I begged to be allowed to die with my family, but because I spoke German they put me in a work group. I had to decide right then, whether to let myself hate the soldiers who had done this. It was an easy decision, really. I was a lawyer. In my practice I had seen too often what hate could do to people's minds and bodies. Hate had just killed the six people who mattered most to me in the world. I decided then that I would spend the rest of my life—whether it was a few days or many years—loving every person I came in contact with."

Wild Bill had watched the family he loved get shot down in cold blood in front of his eyes. Still, he was able to rise above hatred by choosing to love. His choice didn't make the murderers less guilty or less accountable in the overall scheme of things, but it kept him strong and safe in the midst of unthinkable circumstances. His story is a testament to the potential of the human spirit and the power of choosing love over fear. Fear is the opposite of faith. Faith is the inner perception of a reality far more powerful than anything in the external world.

As I tied up the loose ends of my life, the past was becoming resolved, but there was also the present. It was one thing to put former experiences and past relationships to rest but quite another to think about saying good-bye to family and friends currently in my life. I could understand the stories I'd read about people who struggled against impossible odds in order to make it to a special event—a wedding, a holiday, the birth of a child. It was unthinkable that I wouldn't be around for the birth of my third grandchild. The second, Zachary, was not yet a year old, and Matt was now eight. I couldn't imagine not seeing them all grow up.

As a baby Matt had spent a lot of time with me and still loved to spend the night when he could. He had always been delightfully curious and loved to chat about the mysterious nature of life. One night as we made his bed on the floor in my room, I noticed he was unusually quiet. Then he suddenly asked me if it was true that I had cancer.

I hadn't realized until then that no one had spoken to him directly about what was happening to me. I told him that I did have cancer and I didn't know what was going to happen but that I was feeling better all the time. I tried to explain that no one really knows when he or she might die. His little face was serious and he said, "If I were you, I would have that operation." It was another detail he must have overheard.

I didn't know how to answer him. His perception that I wasn't doing all I could touched off a conflict in me. Was I being selfish by making choices that might shorten the time I had with my loved ones? Was I being egotistical in refusing to have an operation that would leave me with a less-than-perfect body? Was I throwing my life away? My rational mind was wreaking havoc and questioning everything I thought I believed: *What ever made me think I could do this my way? Who am I to know what's right?*

Not you, came the response from within as I drifted off to sleep, *but the drop of God within you, your own higher nature.* The words brought a wave of calmness, touching a reality that wasn't clouded by fear or reasoning. My life, my experiences, my beliefs had set me on this path of intuition. This path was part of a plan I believed I had brought into life with me. I believed we all brought in a plan designed to attract a series of personal lessons and direct us toward our unique purpose and life's work.

I slipped into the world of dreams where Matt and I walked over green hills and experienced the world from a grander perspective. I couldn't promise that I would always be around in the flesh. No one can. But I knew we could always walk together here.

6

Making My Way Through the System

Acceptance of one's life has nothing to do with resignation;
it does not mean running away from the struggle. On the
contrary it means accepting it as it comes. . . . To accept
is to say yes to life in its entirety.

PAUL TOURNIER

Along with the challenge of dealing with cancer came the financial realities. When I moved into my little apartment, I applied for supplemental social security and was told it would take a month or two to process the paperwork. I had just enough money to meet my expenses in the meantime.

Three months later my claim still hadn't been completed. When papers to validate my claim had gone to the oncologist, he had written that he suspected I was suicidal because I was refusing the radical treatment that had been offered. Now my claim was being held up pending a psychiatric examination. I was devastated. The oncologist's conclusion was based on one meeting with me under stressful circumstances, and I felt anxious to get the meeting with the psychiatrist over with. A week before the appointment, however, I received a call rescheduling for two weeks later. After a week I received another call for another rescheduling.

I was on an emotional roller coaster, and the stabbing pains in my abdomen grew sharp. I had to do something. I wrote a letter to the agency that was processing my claim and explained that I had a medical diagnosis of advanced cancer and wasn't expected to live long. I was running out of money, and the anticipation of having to comply with a psychiatric examination, ordered because I'd refused radical surgery that would dramatically impact the quality of my life, was compounding an already stressful situation. Whether their agency was going to release funds to me or not, a timely decision would greatly relieve the pressure I was currently under. I ended with a plea to the agency to recognize that in processing claims they were dealing with the lives and emotions of real people.

I wasn't just running out of money—I was out. There were so many ways I already felt like a failure, and now this. I was ashamed to admit that I was out of money and out of options. I applied for welfare and was told to come back in five days. When I went back I was told that I qualified for 120 dollars a month plus food stamps. My stomach scrunched into a knot, and I could barely get any words out. I explained that I lived in the most inexpensive housing in town and even so, 120 dollars wouldn't even pay a third of my rent. The caseworker shrugged her shoulders. I canceled my application for assistance but accepted 50 dollars in food stamps. It was crushing to experience firsthand what some people faced every day. I went to the grocery store on my way home, and when I handed over the food stamps I felt a flush of embarrassment creep up my face.

I didn't know what I was going to do about money, but for the moment I just couldn't think about it. I went to the Letters to God section of my journal and surrendered the situation and all my feelings about it. "I know I'm just one person, God. There are millions of people facing things like this and so much worse."

The next day I got a phone call from a woman at the social security office telling me my appointment with the psychiatrist had been canceled. Tears were stinging my eyes as I asked her when it was being rescheduled for. "No," she said, "it's been canceled. Your claim has been accepted, and you'll be getting retroactive pay from the date of your application four months ago."

An enormous weight was lifted. And now that the social security had come through I was automatically eligible for MediCal, an insurance that pays for health care. It was a relief to know that in case of an emergency I would be able to receive medical care.

Any medical emergency I imagined had to do with the possibility of physical deterioration due to the cancer. But walking home with a bag of groceries in the dusk one evening, I stepped off a curb into a rut and twisted my ankle. I walked the block or two home before I could pull the boot off my swollen foot. It looked like a bad sprain, but I sensed it was broken. I found my MediCal card and called my father to see if he could drive me to the community hospital. When he arrived he said, "That's a sprain all right. I've seen dozens. You don't have to have it X-rayed." But I asked him to take me anyway.

After we waited for two hours, the technician took me in and said, "I've been X-raying bones for twenty years, and I've never called one wrong yet. This is a sprain." A few minutes later he came back with the Xray in hand and a sheepish grin. "Looks like there's always a first time. You cracked an important ankle bone." Then he told me that the doctor who puts on casts wouldn't be in until Wednesday—five days away. I was given crutches and told to keep off my foot until then.

On Wednesday at the clinic, the doctor made a cast from below my knee to my toes. The plaster was hot when she applied it, and I commented that it was good it was the middle of winter and not a hot summer day. She didn't mention that after the chemical reaction of heat the plaster was going to turn ice-cold until it dried—a process that would take twenty-four hours.

That night I couldn't lie down. Every time I tried to, it felt like poison was spreading through my body. My heart raced, my skin crawled, and I was thrown into a panic. The only way I could calm myself was to pace on my crutches in the tiny space of my room. As the hours went by, it got worse.

I called my father at 11 P.M. and asked him to take me to the hospital again. He was groggy from sleep. "My God, what did you do now?" he asked. "Well, I need to get my cast off," I told him. I could imagine him shaking his head, but he didn't say anything. My parents came and drove me to the hospital.

I was embarrassed by the full-blown panic attack I was experiencing. I had to keep moving in order to contain the irrational feeling that I might emotionally explode. I'd had no idea what a panic attack was until then.

It was 1 A.M. before I was called in. The doctor on duty listened as I described the panic I'd been experiencing since the cast was put on. I wanted it off. He said he would prescribe some tranquilizers. My panic heightened. "You don't understand. I have to have this cast off. I don't want tranquilizers. Please! Just take it off."

He tried reason. "The ankle bone is extremely important. It needs to be held in place. It just isn't reasonable to have it out of a cast." Interesting, I thought, that it was OK for the first five days.

My panic worsened. I would take the cast off myself if I could figure out how. Finally, he said he would have to call the attending physician and get permission. I said, "Fine."

"It's now one-thirty in the morning," he said. I agreed that was true.

He walked unhappily to the phone and, when he had my doctor on the line, described my emotional state and my insistence on having the cast off. He had tried to explain to me . . . Then he stopped talking for a minute, and when he started again his tone had completely changed. "Cast claustrophobia? Yes, of course, I'll get it off immediately."

He came back and with serious thoughtfulness explained that when people have cast claustrophobia they absolutely can't wear casts—which was exactly what I'd been trying to tell him. He cut the cast off down the sides and left the underside held on with an ace bandage so it could still support my foot and leg. I could remove it whenever I wanted to.

It worked perfectly. In fact, it was much more sensible than a full cast. I was able to slip it off to take baths, to soak my foot and ankle in Epsom salts, to rub my skin with oil, and to carefully move my muscles so they didn't atrophy during recovery. In five weeks my ankle was X-rayed again, and the doctor was impressed that she couldn't even tell where it had been broken.

With that minor crisis aside I turned my attention to Dr. Turner. For several months she had been urging me to have a pap smear so she could monitor what was going on, but I had kept putting it off. If the test came back positive for cancer, it would nurture the seed in my mind that my cancer was spreading. I knew the danger of self-fulfilling prophecy. I was also aware of the speculation that when a cancer was cut into, as mine had been, cells could be further spread. I consciously worked on holding the perspective that my biopsy had removed a big chunk of the burden and my body was growing strong enough to handle the rest.

Dr. Turner persisted, and out of respect for her support I agreed to have a pap smear. The results came back class 1—normal. I was surprised by my surprise. It felt like a miracle.

But Dr. Turner wasn't satisfied. She wanted to do another colposcopy. I realized that she didn't believe the cancer could be gone. I knew that looking for cancer rather than looking for recovery was a dangerous perspective (you get what you look for), but I thought some good might come out of allowing myself to be studied.

I agreed to have the colposcopy. When I went in, Dr. Turner explained that the results of the pap smear didn't mean much, as new cells grow over the opening. The test didn't indicate what was going on at a deeper level. Now, instead of the colposcopy, she wanted to do a more invasive procedure, called an ECC.

Alarm bells sounded. I wanted to leave, but I didn't know how to do that without seeming rude or irrational. I stayed for the test. I was told the results would take a week. Three weeks later I had made four calls to the office and was finally told that Dr. Turner wouldn't be in until the following Friday. The receptionist wouldn't release the test results to me.

I remembered that the results from the breast biopsy had been given to me over the phone, but the results of the cervical biopsy that showed cancer had been withheld until an office visit. Were they deliberately not giving me bad news again? I had almost another week to wait and could feel the tension building up. At night I found it hard to sleep.

On Friday the doctor's office called to say that Dr. Turner wanted to consult with another doctor before talking to me, and it might be another week before I could get the results. My chest was pounding. If the test had shown no cancer, I was sure she would have told me outright.

I waited another week and Dr. Turner finally called. All cells were normal, she told me, but her voice didn't match the good news. Then she said she had conferred with three pathologists and two gynecologists who all agreed that the tests didn't mean anything. They had all advised her not to put me through further tests. There was no way to monitor the cancer, which could be anywhere by now.

My relief at hearing that the cells were normal was quickly displaced by disappointment. The conferring doctors had all discounted the test results. Doubts crept into my mind. Over the next few days my energy fell dramatically and the pains in my abdomen sharpened.

I was in the middle of an experience that left me feeling isolated from the rest of the world. I knew of some cancer groups, but because I wasn't receiving conventional treatment I hesitated to join one. I didn't want to be discouraged by any more invalidation about my choices. But it was a lonely road, and I decided to meet with the group at the community hospital to give it a try.

I entered a large room where tables had been pushed together end to end to form a long rectangle. As I slid into a cold metal chair, quizzical faces nodded and smiled in my direction. Swollen, pale, the faces were captivating. One was especially thin under the dome of a bald head. My eyes glanced at hands that were wrapped around cans of Coke and Pepsi. In the middle of the table was a large square cake, the white frosting thick and dotted with sugary flowers of pink and yellow and green. Plates of cookies lined both sides.

The woman across from me introduced herself as a nurse and held up a metal pitcher. "Would anyone like coffee?" she asked. "We have regular and unleaded!" "I'll take the real thing," laughed the too-thin man with the shining bald head. She passed it down. "Welcome to the cancer support group. . . ."

I was tremendously moved by the struggles of the individuals sitting around that table, but I couldn't relate to the unquestioning acceptance that the attending physician's opinion was the only one that mattered. No one seemed to question the treatments that were recommended or to consider diet or lifestyle changes or to factor the effects of emotions into their disease. There was no mention of how cancer feeds on the kind of sugary treats that decorated the table.

I was especially bothered by what seemed to be the view that cancer is a random event that attacks certain victims for no particular reason, and that there is nothing we could personally do about it. I was determined not to be a victim. Indeed, I was determined to make sense out of this experience. I went home still feeling alone but resolved to continue to meet cancer in my own way. Whatever came, I would act from my inner sense of guidance, one step at a time.

I was back at the hospital a few nights later, on November fifth. At noon Nathaniel James Marshall was born. I brought Matthew and Zachary to the delivery room to meet their new brother. Zachary snuggled up on my lap and buried his face in my chest. He wasn't ready yet to see the wrinkled little baby that we were all so excited about. For a moment Randy put Nathan in my free arm, and I held both boys close. It was a milestone for me. I had made it this far.

More than a year after my diagnosis I was feeling good, taking long walks, and living with more energy during the day. I felt it was time to have a general exam and pap test, but I didn't want to return to the doctor who didn't really believe I could get well.

I decided to make an appointment with my daughter's doctor. Cindy had told her about me, and Dr. Lynch had been genuinely interested and positive. Every time she saw Cindy she asked for an update on how I was doing and applauded my progress. I called the office and made an appointment.

At the clinic I went to the check-in desk for new patients and filled out all the forms. The receptionist read them over and noted that I didn't have insurance. I told her I was paying cash, and she said that was fine. Then I mentioned that I had a MediCal card but wasn't planning to use it. She looked nervous and excused herself. Another woman came to the desk and told me that there had been a mistake, and I wouldn't be able to see Dr. Lynch. People on MediCal had to go to the community hospital. "But I'm not using MediCal," I told her, sure there was some misunderstanding. "I'm paying cash." Her manner became curt, and she asked if I'd like to see the patient advocate. Assuming there was just some misunderstanding, I said yes. I was directed to another waiting room and a call was made. I could see two receptionists looking in my direction sympathetically.

A tall woman in spiked heels brusquely approached me a few minutes later and asked if I was Cheryl Canfield. Without identifying herself she said she would bring Mr. Black to talk to me. I assumed Mr. Black was the patient advocate. She came back with an impeccably dressed man who extended his hand and identified himself as the director of the clinic. This man then waved the woman, evidently the patient advocate, away.

He told me that the medical center didn't see people who were on MediCal. I repeated that I was paying cash. He said I could see a doctor at the community center. I told him I had come specifically to see Dr. Lynch because she was interested in my case and I had a great deal of confidence in the things I'd heard about her. I reminded him I was paying cash. He became obviously annoyed and waved me away, saying, "Go to the community center. You're done here."

I was stunned and stood there looking at him. Out of the corner of my eye I could see the receptionists listening sympathetically and shaking their heads. Looking exasperated Mr. Black continued, "It's a privilege to be served at this clinic, not a right. You're not welcome here."

His words felt sharper than a slap. I couldn't talk. I felt ashamed of my naiveté. Tears were collecting behind my eyes, ready to burst loose, but I held them back, not wanting to be further embarrassed. I turned and walked away, carrying the weight of humiliation. *So this is what discrimination feels like*, I thought.

When I got home I cried until I exhausted myself. I knew that what had happened to me was minor compared to what has been done, and continues to be done, to whole groups of minorities. I wanted to be strong enough to confront and try to change the system—or at the very least stop the director of the clinic from treating anyone else in that way. I could have gone to the clinic board or written an article or gone to a local news reporter. I didn't. At that time, I couldn't even muster up the courage or the energy to deal with Mr. Black, much less confront the whole system.

But I did get in to see Dr. Lynch. She gave my daughter instructions for me on how to bypass the front desk. When I saw her she examined me thoroughly and took a lengthy history. She commended me for the strength of my convictions. While taking a pap smear she described the tissues she was observing as pink and healthy and praised me overall for the excellent shape I was in. When I came back for the results, she said they were perfectly normal. I told her that my previous doctor and her colleagues had believed that the tests were meaningless. Matter-of-factly, she stated, "Well, I say if it doesn't show cancer, you don't have cancer."

It was amazing to hear those words and to feel them sinking in. I drove to Cindy's house to tell her the news, and Zachary came running down the hallway, throwing himself into my arms. I caught him and was swinging him around when Cindy came into sight. "Be careful, he weighs a ton!" she exclaimed, and eyed me carefully. "You must be feeling pretty good."

I told her the results from the test and what the doctor had said. "Do you think you're in remission?" she asked hopefully. "Oh no," I laughed. "Remission sounds like there's something hanging over my shoulder waiting to pounce. I don't know what's going to happen tomorrow or next year. I only know that today I'm well."

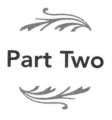

Part Two

Life Stories

7

The Spiritual Path

*You cannot really know with your limited intelligence or with
your five senses that there is more than the physical universe—
but when you awaken the divine nature, it knows.*

PEACE PILGRIM

The quest to discover "Who am I?" and "Why am I here?" is often preceded by some crisis that serves as a wake-up call and has the potential to propel us, if we're willing, into a more expanded or spiritual awareness. It was the Vietnam war, many years prior to the cancer, that first led me into a spiritual search; but it was cancer that gave me the opportunity to test the principles I had come to believe in. Would I have the courage and faith to live my beliefs through this difficult challenge? I felt compelled to look back on the journey that had brought me to this point.

I grew up in a family that went to church every Sunday and accepted certain exclusive beliefs. From a very young age I realized that many of my young friends fell outside of the guidelines that were outlined by the church as necessary for salvation. It was a troublesome awareness; I consoled myself by thinking that I would understand when I was older. But as I got older I realized that such beliefs were more human than divine, and I left the confines of formal religion. I knew there was a guiding force in my life, but I didn't try to define it.

By the mid-seventies I was married to a Vietnam veteran and raising a young daughter. Stories of the atrocities that had taken place in Vietnam came home with the physically and psychologically wounded young men and took a toll on my generation. There was a general numbing that found expression in the saying, "God is dead." Many men like my husband, who had survived physically, were looking for a way to escape the nightmares that screamed out in the dark hours or slipped out in haunting memories during the day.

Andy called me his window to the world. Although I couldn't really understand how devastating his experiences had been, I felt the heaviness he carried. There was an indefinable void around him, or perhaps a wall through which he wasn't able to fully connect with the world.

In the aftermath of the war we struggled with our inner battles, trying but failing to find some way to reconcile the atrocities of war with a deeper sense that humankind was intended for something far better. While we accumulated the external security that served as a measurement of success, internally I felt like a rudderless ship tossing about randomly on vast ocean currents. Where was my direction? Just when I had given up hope of ever finding an answer, it came in the form of a completely unexpected and pivotal inner experience.

THE FOREST VISION

Andy, ten-year-old Cindy, and I had driven to a state park in northern California to meet Andy's coworkers and their families for a Fourth of July picnic celebration. As we drove into the park in the early morning, I noticed a halolike radiance around the bushes at the entrance, and even the bird fluttering alongside the car seemed to be emanating light. I didn't make much of it at first, assuming it was just a reflection of the morning sun. But as we got out and started walking along a shaded path underneath the giant trees, I realized that everything in sight had this beautiful light emanation. There were even flecks of gold in the air.

As we walked along I noticed that all of my senses had become extraordinarily keen. Sounds picked up by my ears were instantly translated into images in my mind's eye of a squirrel or the hooves of a deer or a bird hopping through the dense brush. Whatever it was, I could see it clearly in my inner vision. I was drawn into the rhythm around me; it seemed that the trees and even the air swelled and emptied with my breath.

My consciousness shifted, and for a time it seemed I was somewhere else. I can best describe it as walking into another dimension in which I was not conscious of my physical body or surroundings, but at the same time extremely conscious of many impressions. The spiritual nature of reality became clear and obvious, as though this awareness had been tucked behind some curtain that was suddenly pulled open.

Just as suddenly, I was drawn into a scene just before my birth:

I'm watching a young woman I recognize to be me, although she looks somewhat different than I currently look, sitting in a garden where flowers are blooming in exquisite colors. The environment is softer and it replicates the physical world, except that everything seems intensified. Colors are more brilliant and sounds more pure, although words can scarcely describe it. As I survey the scene I'm flooded with recollections.

This garden is where the young woman and others gather to listen to the one who is called the teacher. Time here isn't divided into night and day as it is in the physical dimension where the teacher now resides, even though she has graduated from the lessons of that denser plane, the place where memory fades and time is lived from the perspective that life begins at birth and ends at death. She is able now to enter an awakened state even while on that plane, having chosen to be born into a physical body in order to help others break through the forgetfulness of the earth experience and wake up to the collective lessons of nonviolence and compassion, before the technological advancements of an as yet immature society render the earth school uninhabitable.

While her body of flesh rests during the night hours on the physical plane, the teacher appears in the garden to counsel souls from all the surrounding villages as they prepare for the continuance of their journey into the physical world. When they enter the flesh their true identities will be forgotten, and they will face the tasks they set out for themselves without memory of having chosen them. It will be both a great challenge and a great opportunity for much growth.

"Remember," she is saying, "when the time comes to choose from the lessons you have left to learn, you will choose only those that you yourself decide to take on. The more you choose to learn, the more difficult it will seem, and you will not know why it is that such difficulties come to you. If you persevere and work successfully through each lesson at hand, the growth you attain will permit you to penetrate another veil in the shroud of forgetfulness. The time will come when your vision will be clear and even in the physical world your true identity will emerge and become your reality.

"It takes a good deal of courage to take on the lessons that still await you. The more timid among you will take on one or two, and that is fine. But if you have the courage to take on several and work through all of them, you will have made that much more progress in your journey and will require fewer excursions into the world of physical experience.

"The earth life is alluring, and without memory its illusion is strong. One of the most difficult illusions to break through is the illusion of separation. Here you know that you are not separate from one another or from God, the creative Source that runs through all things and binds all things together. Even while in a physical body, once you penetrate this veil you will know from within that you are never alone. You are always accompanied by spirit guides from the angelic realm and teachers who have themselves walked the earth plane. But when you are born into a body of flesh, you will forget. Your guides will be most able to reach you when your minds are still in meditation or sleep.

"There is another illusion that causes much confusion. Identifying yourself as the body, rather than that which activates the body, creates a sense of limitation. The forgetfulness that is a condition of the

physical world creates the belief that it is only through physical form that you create and think and have your being. The truth that you create your physical form and its condition in accordance with your thoughts and emotions is lost. The knowledge that you are spiritual beings attempting to learn important lessons and to find the unique work you have set out to undertake while in the flesh can only be found in the quiet stillness within. There, in that inner sanctuary, lies the truth. It is always with you.

"There are many adventures awaiting you in the physical world. If you make it through the veil of forgetfulness to the heart of truth, the privilege of consciously creating the conditions of your experiences awaits you. Your potential to create, even while in the flesh, is unlimited. If you err and create only material gain, accumulating for yourself without regard to others, you will reap a basket of lessons to return to again and again. Irresponsible actions that in any way exploit or violate another create a deficit, which unchecked will eventually lead to a bankruptcy of the soul.

"Nothing binds one to suffering more than this. You are accountable for every thought, every action, every feeling you send out. There is no judgment in this. Universal law applies to everyone equally. Living in harmony with these laws is the path that will bring you into conscious awareness of your spiritual nature.

"Remember this: the supreme law is the law of love. No matter how strong the illusion, when love is put aside for fear or greed, and when violence, whether emotional or physical, is done by you to another, that violence is done to your own soul and you carry it with you.

"The earth life is like a dream. Violence done to your body only removes you from the dream. Violence done by you to another ties you not only to the dream but to the experience of violence over and over again, to be played out by you both as victim and perpetrator."

When the teacher is gone the girl remains in the garden, gazing into the distance. She is joined by the one she calls her brother. The members of the family in this village, as in others, learn and grow in constellation with one another. In and out of the land of dreams they come together, sharing in one another's joys and sorrows and learning about love in all its levels and expressions. The nature of the relationships often changes on the physical side so that a sibling in one life might be a daughter or close friend in another. On the side between dreams, ethereal forms, although fine in vibration, resemble the image of the body most recently inhabited.

The brother stands tall with a slender frame and fine, chiseled features. His eyes, most often radiating a youthful sense of fun, study the girl. "You're thinking about leaving, aren't you?" he asks. Although time here isn't perceived in the same strung-out linear way as in the physical world, progression is noted in the movement of events and the entering and leaving of members of the community.

"Yes," she responds. "I'm being called to enter the physical world. The guardian is waiting for me. She and the caretaker will be my parents. For some time now we have been communicating during those periods when their bodies are at rest."

The guardian has already taken the role in the family as well as in the greater community of providing emotional support to the various members. She and the girl have been together in many different relationships, and their bond is close. The guardian, who is to be the girl's mother when she enters the world of flesh, is now in a physical form not unlike that of her previous one, as the body merely reflects consciousness, and changes in appearance evolve with the same methodical development as changes in personality and emotion and intellect. She is of small frame with delicate hands and feet, reflecting an earlier life in the Orient. Her sweetness of nature and stability of emotions are also reflections of that long-ago life; these qualities have further been nurtured in subsequent periods.

The caretaker, who is to be the girl's father, used to tend the village gardens with devoted attention. Having a perceptive sense of how things fit together to become functional, he also often conversed with the inventors whose advancements moved evolution forward. He is of average build and moves with deliberation, ever focused on the execution of some task. Of temperament he is sensitive, not prone to light chatter *but fixed on the nature of things. His big hands are almost always busy organizing clutter into orderliness or turning some broken thing into something useful.*

The brother's eyes deepen at the girl's words, and she looks lovingly at him. "It won't be long. You'll know when the time is right for you to come."

As the girl makes her way to the hall of preparation, she meets a cousin. He is tall, with a gaunt face, and his deep-set brown eyes convey sadness. On his right temple a mole marks the spot where a bullet entered during a battle, shortening his previous life and leaving him bewildered. Both the girl and the cousin are being called to journey to the physical world once again. Each will take a list of lessons yet to be learned, both their own individual lessons and those to be considered on a collective level.

The cousin reaches into the vessel in front of him and with determination draws out several slips. After speaking with him, the wise ones nod and give him their blessings. The girl's eyes meet the cousin's and she smiles encouragement; then he is gone.

The girl peers into the vessel in front of her. She hesitates before drawing out several slips. They contain major lessons of both personal and collective consequence. The council of learned ones speaks kindly to her.

"In the journey of your soul the time has come to expand the riches of your inner experience into the outer world of expression. You are entering at a time of great need in the area of collective transformation and spiritual awakening. There is a great struggle between forces that would lead to great destruction and annihilation and forces that would lead to a golden age of peace.

"Collectively, humanity has reached a crossroads, and the outcome lies in the balance. In order for peace to prevail, conflict and oppression must be overcome. In order for love to prevail, hatred and prejudice must be overcome. In order for wisdom to prevail, ignorance and fear must be overcome. The lessons are personal as well as collective, and every individual is helping to determine the course of human evolution."

The wise one now speaking pauses, placing his hand gently on her

forehead, and then continues softly. "Take heart. The teacher will be
with you there as here, and through your own effort your path will cross
with hers as you are ready. There is much you will remember. The
guides and teachers are with humanity in abundance during this time
of great transition. Remember that one person in alignment with God
can have more force than an army.

"The way to discover your soul's journey in the life ahead will be to
awaken to the reality within. To find your strength you will confront
your weaknesses. You will need to pass through the dark night in order
to penetrate the veil. Do you wish to take these lessons on now?" The
girl nods her assent.

As the image receded I found myself back in the forest, Andy,
Cindy, and I all walking along a trail in unusual silence. I felt a lingering sensation of having been in an altered state. It was like awakening from a bout of amnesia with the forgotten details of my
identity flooding in. When I walked out of the woods that day, my
perception of the world and of myself had completely changed. I
could never go back to the unconscious level of functioning that had
been my life.

RAPID CHANGES

When we returned to the picnic area, a half dozen or so barbecue pits
were lit. Hot dogs and hamburgers and steaks were thrown on the
grills, and as the odors wafted by I was startled by the smell of roast-
ing flesh. When the steak I had brought was put on my plate, I saw
the animal that it had been and couldn't eat it. I had always known
that I would never kill an animal or a bird or even a fish, and now it
seemed strange that I had ever considered eating them. No one I
knew was a vegetarian. I had no idea what to eat in place of meat, yet
I was certain that I would never knowingly eat flesh again. (It was a
delightful surprise, as I later did the research, to find that it was actually healthy to eat a diet based on grains and legumes and vegetables
and fruit.)

The next big change came a few weeks later when Andy came home from a physical exam. He had gone to a doctor because of pains in his chest and was told that he was allergic to cigarette smoke. He didn't smoke but I did. I knew that smoke was hazardous to smokers, but at that time there was little talk about the effects of secondhand smoke.

Upon hearing the news, I needed a cigarette so I went outside. I sat in the backyard watching the smoke curl upward in an alluring spiral. Smoking was connected to everything I did. Whenever the phone rang, for instance, I picked up a cigarette before I answered it. I now looked at the wall beside me, wondering if a hole could be drilled to run a phone cord outside. I also enjoyed smoking in bed at night when I was reading a good book, but from now on, I thought, I would have to go outside. What if it was raining? I looked up and imagined extending the roof out to make a covered patio.

A light broke through the smoke-filled recesses of my mind: cigarettes were governing my life! Here I was planning to remodel my house in order to accommodate my habit. The idea was shocking.

Never again, I thought. *I refuse to be a slave to this stick of nicotine!* I threw the cigarette to the ground and stomped it out. I fully expected to go through withdrawal and experience the cravings I'd always felt when I'd quit smoking before, but it didn't happen. I even forgot about the cigarettes I had pushed to the back of the refrigerator "in case of emergency" until months later, when I pulled out the vegetable bin while cleaning and found the moldy pack.

These outer lifestyle changes represented only a part of the amazing metamorphosis in my inner life. I had been living in a little box comprised of the people and things I was familiar with. Now there was a whole new world of ideas to explore. I started reading voraciously, but instead of the usual novels and adventure stories my interest turned to philosophy and art, comparative religions and psychology. There was hardly anything I wasn't interested in. I had come to realize that there was more to this existence than "seeking the good life," and my mind was like a thirsty sponge soaking up information.

When I read about an organization called the Theosophical Society, I was drawn by the group's purpose, which was to encourage the study of comparative religions, science, and the powers latent in humankind. What particularly attracted me was their motto: "There is no religion higher than Truth." The national headquarters in Wheaton, Illinois, housed a staff of forty in a beautiful setting of trees and gardens. The forces calling me there were strong, and I had no intention of resisting.

8

Encounter with a Modern Mystic:
A Woman Called Peace Pilgrim

The universe is a school where people will eventually
develop into the image and likeness of God.
It will exist as long as a school is needed.

PEACE PILGRIM

Within months following my experience in the forest, Andy and Cindy and I were packing up to drive from California to the Theosophical Society in Wheaton, Illinois. When I first brought up the possibility of our actually going there to work and study, I was surprised at how receptive Andy was to the idea. I took it to be like-mindedness at the time, although in retrospect I suspect it had more to do with his own shattered identity since Vietnam; he looked to me to interpret the world and give our lives direction. Almost immediately we were caught up in plans to move.

We put an ad in the paper for our house and signed the mortgage over to the first couple who came to see it. We called the Salvation Army and asked them to send over a large truck to take away the furniture in our four-bedroom house. Then we packed our remaining belongings, mostly clothes and necessities, into our green Pontiac, and the three of us headed east along with Cindy's small dog, Li'l Bit. The car died in the salt flats just outside of Salt Lake

City. When we drove into the Theosophical Society, it was in a rented van.

In the excitement of our bold move we hadn't thought to let anyone know we were coming, and our arrival created quite a stir. After a hastily called meeting, a decision was made to take us in, but there was no place to put us. The individual houses on the property were already occupied by families. The three-story main building housed forty adults and included several offices, a formal library, and an auditorium. The basement included a kitchen and dining room, where everyone gathered for meals and recreation. Neither dogs nor children were allowed to live in the main building.

The next day an apartment was rented for us within walking distance. We were to take our meals with everyone else, and both Andy and I would receive twenty-five dollars a week in exchange for work. He was placed in maintenance, and I became Miriam's assistant in housekeeping.

It wasn't long after our arrival in Wheaton that I heard about a woman who would be coming to stay at the Theosophical Society for several weeks while she was speaking in the Chicago area. This unusual woman, who called herself Peace Pilgrim, had been walking around the United States for twenty-three years. She was much sought after as a speaker; her engagements were booked and her itinerary planned years in advance. She considered herself a religious pilgrim, carried no money and didn't accept any, and owned only the clothes on her back. She had made a vow to walk until humanity learned the ways of peace, and she accepted shelter and food only when it was offered. She never asked. The moment I heard about her I knew I was about to come face to face with my teacher.

THE BIG MOMENT ARRIVES

The first time I saw her she was coming through the large arch that framed the entrance to the grounds. I watched her from a grove of trees, content for the moment to observe her from a distance. Her stride was long and confident, exuding a sense of purpose. This moment endures in my memory like a clear photograph.

That night she spoke to a small intimate group in the formal oak library. Her silver hair was caught up in a ponytail that bounced to the animated rhythm of her words. I was struck as much by her energy as by the amazing stories she told. She was obviously a senior, her shining face creased with wrinkles, but her answer to the question of her age was, "I'm ageless and in radiant health."

If judged by appearance alone, she would have been easy to dismiss as some kind of nut. Her clothes were navy blue from her worn canvas sneakers up to the tailored shirt she wore beneath a faded blue tunic. The tunic bore large white letters that proclaimed her name on the front and "25,000 MILES ON FOOT FOR PEACE" on the back.

She wore the lettered tunic so that those who were curious could approach her to find out what her message was about. "You're in a much better position to speak to people when they approach you than when you approach them. And the most interesting people come. They either have a lively curiosity or are genuinely interested in the cause of peace."

From this first introduction I was struck by her simple profundity. The words she spoke brought deepening clarity to principles I wanted to believe in but hadn't fully comprehended. I also marveled at her level of personal simplicity. The pockets that went all around the bottom of her tunic held everything Peace owned, which included a comb, toothbrush, maps, pen, and any unanswered mail. "Gandhi didn't carry a toothbrush or a comb," someone pointed out. With a deep, hearty laugh she said, "He didn't have hair or teeth!"

Peace spoke unself-consciously, completely absorbed in relating her story. She had taken her name when she started her pilgrimage so that when people remembered her they would be reminded of her message and not her personality. "People can only remember so much, and I want them to remember the important things."

She struck me as the most authentic individual I'd ever met; yet despite the realness she was shrouded in a kind of mystery. The only name she gave was Peace Pilgrim, and she wouldn't tell her age, saying with conviction that she remained ageless by putting age out of her mind.

She had been crisscrossing the country on foot for more than two decades, counting more than twenty-five thousand miles in the first ten years. Her walking was her occupation; she called it her retirement project. She had started out with great determination and courage during the McCarthy era, when war was raging in Korea and congressional committees considered people guilty until proven innocent. It was a time when there was a great deal of fear and it was safest to be apathetic. It was easy to imagine that she had walked out of nowhere, an apparition meant to wake people up from their apathy and get them thinking.

She talked about what she called the whole peace picture, "peace among nations, peace between groups and individuals, peace with the environment, and that very important inner peace, which is where peace begins." In her message to us that first night she talked about a period in her life that she called her spiritual growing up:

> There were hills and valleys in that spiritual growing up period. Then in the midst of the struggle there came a wonderful mountaintop experience—the first glimpse of what the life of inner peace was like. That came when I was out walking in the early morning. All of a sudden I felt more uplifted than I had ever been. I knew timelessness and spacelessness and lightness. I did not seem to be walking on the earth. There were no people or even animals around, but every flower, every bush, every tree seemed to wear a halo. There was a light emanation around everything and flecks of gold fell like slanted rain through the air.
>
> This is sometimes called the illumination period. The most important part of it was the realization of the oneness of all creation. Not only all human beings—I knew that all human beings were one. But now I knew also a oneness with the rest of creation.

The creatures that walk the earth and the growing things of the earth. The air, the water, the earth itself. And most wonderful of all, a oneness with that which permeates all and binds all together and gives life to all. A oneness with that which many would call God.*

Tears stung my eyes as her story gave confirmation to what I had experienced. Everything else disappeared and I was alone in the audience as Peace spoke. The concepts she espoused, like the vision that had come to me in the forest, were so familiar that even though I was hearing them for the first time, I already knew them. Her words were stirring awake parts of me that had been slumbering.

The message of her pilgrimage was, Overcome evil with good, falsehood with truth, and hatred with love. "There's nothing new in the message," she said. "The Golden Rule would do as well. The key word for our time is *practice.*" For the duration of the time that Peace was in the area, I went to hear her speak several times a week. She spoke at colleges and universities and various local groups. She gave the sermon at several church services, including a Catholic mass, and was interviewed on radio and television.

Before embarking on her pilgrimage Peace had gone through a process that she called her steps toward inner peace. Without that, she said, she wouldn't have been able to walk as she did, on faith. At some of her talks, especially in college psychology classes, she would draw a chart as seen on page 65 outlining the steps she had taken:

You have free will as to whether you will finish the mental and emotional growing up. Many choose not to. You have free will as to whether you will begin the spiritual growing up. The beginning of it is the time when you feel completely willing, without

---

*Friends of Peace Pilgrim, *Peace Pilgrim: Her Life and Work in her Own Words.* (Santa Fe: Ocean Tree Books, 1982). EDITOR'S NOTE: All Peace Pilgrim quotes appearing in this book are attributable to the citation above and/or the author's first-hand experience.

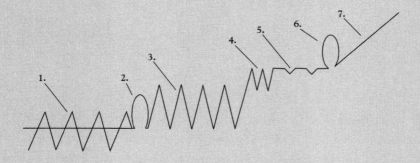

1. The first stage of life is characterized by the ups and downs of emotion that we experience when our lives are governed by the self-centered nature. The body, mind, and emotions are all instruments that can be used by the self-centered nature but never fully controlled, because the self-centered nature is itself controlled by wishes for comfort and convenience on the part of the body, by demands of the mind, and by outbursts of emotions. The struggle here is between the body, mind, and emotions and the self-centered nature. At this point life is very much governed by early training and beliefs that have been programmed into the subconscious mind.

2. Unlike physical growth, which happens automatically, and mental and emotional growing up, which most people do to some degree, spiritual growth requires a conscious choice. It begins with a complete willingness, without reservation, to leave the self-centered life and begin to work for the good of the whole. It is the first point of no return.

3. During this period there is a recognition of what psychologists refer to as *ego* and *conscience*. It's as though we have two selves or two natures with two different viewpoints. Because the viewpoints are so different, there can be struggle during this period between the two selves, the lower and the higher self, with many hills and valleys.

4. This is the peak or illumination experience, a high enough rise in consciousness to look at the universe through the eyes of the higher nature. It is the first glimpse of inner peace. "I have never felt separate since."

5. During this period long plateaus of inner peace are experienced, but there are still times when we slip out of harmony. "I could return again and again to this wonderful mountaintop, and then I could stay there for longer and longer periods of time and just slip out occasionally. "

6. During this period the spiritual growth pattern is completed, and inner peace is attained. The higher nature has taken over and fully controls the body, mind, and spirit. This is another point of no return. The struggle is over now because we will do the right thing, and we don't need to be pushed into it. "I knew that for me the struggle was over, that finally I had succeeded in giving my life or finding inner peace."

7. In this final stage learning and growing continue, but there is no longer a struggle.

any reservations, to leave the self-centered life. And most choose not to. But it was doing that growth and finding inner peace that prepared me for the pilgrimage I walk today.

It's as though the central figure of the jigsaw of your life is complete and clear and unchanging, and around the edges other pieces keep fitting in. There is always a growing edge but the progress is harmonious. There is a feeling of always being surrounded by all of the good things, like love and peace and joy. It seems like a protective surrounding, and there is an unshakeableness within which takes you through any situation you may need to face.

You are now in control of your life. I can say to my body, "Lie down there on that cement floor and go to sleep," and it obeys. I can say to my mind, "Shut out everything else and concentrate on the job before you," and it is obedient. I can say to my emotions, "Be still, even in the face of this terrible situation," and they are still. A great philosopher has said, *He who seems to be out of step may be following a different drummer.* And now you are following a different drummer: the higher nature instead of the lower nature.

Peace felt that we all have a special job in life, but because we have free will we don't always seek it out. She taught that every one of us comes into this life with a unique purpose, which can only be found in the stillness within. Walking a pilgrimage, she conceded, was an unusual calling. Most of us are called to simple everyday occupations that serve a useful purpose in society and that we enjoy doing.

Very often, as children, we are more aware of that inner voice, and because we haven't yet developed rational thinking we don't question it. As we get older it fades or gets lost periodically in the busyness and distraction of growing up. It is most often in the quiet of prayer or meditation that I now find it, or in moments of personal crisis. Crisis, which the Chinese pictogram depicts as both danger and opportunity, can function as an abrupt wake-up call. What shakes us up tends to wake us up and get our attention.

Peace saw the Earth life as a school—a place where we have an opportunity to learn and grow. What distinguishes humans from the other life forms around us is an ongoing evolution of the soul on its journey of spiritual growth and a recognition of the invisible reality within—what she called the divine nature. Because we have free will, people are in varied stages of growth, she would say; we will continue to experience human lives until we have fully claimed our spiritual divinity and transcended the ego or self-centered nature.

As Peace walked into the sixties, seventies, and early eighties she continued to assert that we are living in a period of great transition, with strong forces pushing toward chaos. All of us who are alive today have an influence on the outcome. We have free will to choose to do nothing—allowing violent forces to push us toward destruction—or to choose to stand with uncompromising courage to overcome hatred with love.

9

Peace Pilgrim on Healing

There are two types of healing, whether it is physical healing or otherwise. One is removal of cause, which is good. The other is removal of symptom, which merely postpones the reckoning.

PEACE PILGRIM

Peace recognized all experiences that come to people as opportunities to learn and grow. Healing, whether mental or physical or emotional, is the same—an opportunity for more learning and growth.

"If only you could see the whole picture," she taught, "if you knew the whole story, you would realize that no problem ever comes to you that does not have a purpose in your life. When you perceive this you will recognize that problems are opportunities in disguise. If you did not face problems you would just drift through life. It is in solving problems in accordance with the highest light we have that inner growth is attained."

Peace described spiritual healing as the removal of cause; this motivates us to solve whatever problems life sets before us. Psychic healing is the removal of symptoms and only temporary. If a symptom is removed, she said, it will either manifest again or another symptom will come in its place. I was surprised when she said she would never put her hands on people who were ill or pray for their recovery. Instead she prayed that an individual's life come into harmony with

God's will. Faith can move mountains, Peace agreed, but her prayer was that cause be removed, so healing would be permanent.

Spiritual healing is not always as spectacular as the removal of symptoms, she cautioned, because it may take time to learn the lesson contained therein; but physical healing often follows. At other times certain conditions are part of a person's life plan, as in the case of a woman Peace told us about.

The woman was thirty years old when Peace met her. She was bitter because she had been born crippled. Her parents were well-off financially and had sent her to the best schools, but she constantly compared herself to her sister, who was very attractive and had a more or less perfect body.

Peace asked the young woman if she believed there was life after the Earth life and she said yes. Then Peace asked her if she could consider that the soul might have had experience before the Earth life. The young woman began to protest the idea, so Peace asked her to just sleep on it. In the morning the woman had decided that it was just as logical to think that there is something before as after. Soon she accepted the idea that we live in an orderly universe, that cause-and-effect also applied in the condition she had been born with, and she lost her bitterness.

"I saw the woman spiritually healed, but without being physically healed," Peace told us, "and I finally discovered why. The last I saw of her she was joyously teaching crippled children. What a wonderful inspiration she was to them, as I could never be because I am in a whole body. When a handicap is accepted, it stops being a problem, and the person becomes a beautiful inspiration to the people around them."

THE EAGER BEAVER PSYCHIC HEALER

Peace cautioned those in the healing arts to help others find their own spiritual healing, the removal of cause, and not the removal of symptoms. In the beginning, she said, many of us don't realize the difference and become "eager beaver psychic healers."

Let's say I am a psychic healer living next door to you and you have chosen to come into this life to face some kind of physical symptom until you have removed the cause. Well, when the symptom manifests, I remove it. And so the symptom manifests again and I then remove it again, and I manage to keep that symptom removed.

When you step over to the disembodied side of life for another reason altogether, instead of blessing me for having removed the symptom you'll say, "That meddler! I came to solve this problem but she kept removing the symptom and therefore I never solved it!"

When one meddles in the life of another it will just cause the symptoms not only to re-manifest, but carry over into another lifetime. Most healers do not know this and they go on removing symptoms. With God's help you can solve the problem and any other problem that life sets before you.

If you are able to put your life completely into God's hands, with a genuine acceptance of God's will, whatever it might be—physical healing may come, and spiritual healing will certainly come. Healing doesn't always mean staying on this side of life. Sometimes God has other plans for us—and both sides are really one.

WORKING ON CAUSE

Shortly after Peace Pilgrim left Wheaton, my mother called to tell me that she had found a lump in one of her breasts. It wasn't the first time. Several years earlier she had grown a lump in her right breast that had been surgically removed. The lump was benign. Within two years of that, a lump had grown in her left breast. Again it had been removed and was found to be benign. A third time a lump had grown in her breast and was removed. I had been with her in the recovery room when she woke up that last time, and she had been terrified that she had lost her breast. She had not. The lump had been precancerous, and a lumpectomy had been done with no further treatment necessary. Now a lump was growing once again.

"The doctor keeps cutting them out," my mother told me, "but my body keeps growing them. It's obvious that my body is going to continue growing lumps until whatever it is that's causing them changes, and in the meantime these growths are progressing toward cancer. I'm not going to go under the knife again. There must be something I can do to change this pattern."

I told her Peace's story about the eager beaver psychic healer, and she felt a similarity with her own situation. Her lumps had been surgically removed again and again but nothing was being done about the cause.

My mother and I brainstormed about what she might do to try to help herself. I remembered hearing Peace talk about fasting as a method for dissolving tumors that were not yet cancerous. She had said that a twenty-four- or thirty-six-hour fast once every week, drinking only distilled water, was just as effective and not so difficult as a long fast. Mom liked the idea and began at once.

She and I were beginning to understand that the body is inextricably connected with the mind and emotions, and that if something is out of balance in one, the others are also affected. We became detectives trying to unravel a mystery; we considered all the possibilities.

We suspected that the use of pesticides in food sources might be a contributing factor and my mother started removing anything from her diet that was known or thought to contribute to breast cancer. She stopped drinking tea because of the caffeine. She had already eliminated red meat and fowl, and now she gave up fish.

She initiated a quiet time each day to be introspective and pay attention to emotions that might be coming up for her. For instance, she realized that although her children were grown she still worried about us and took on our problems. She started reframing her perspective to recognize that, while it was appropriate to offer her support, it was time to cut the strings and trust that we were capable of learning our own lessons.

She continued to go to her doctor periodically to monitor the lump. At first he said, "Well, it doesn't seem to have grown." Then he began saying, "It seems to be a little smaller. I don't know what you're doing, but keep it up!" Alternatives to Western medicine and body-mind connections weren't generally given serious consideration in the seventies, so she was reluctant to share her strategy with the doctor. Within months the lump was gone altogether. In more than twenty years it hasn't returned.

10

The Journey Home

Two roads diverged in a wood, and I—I took the one least traveled by, and that has made all the difference.

ROBERT FROST

After a year at the Theosophical Society we felt the time had come to move on, taking what we had learned into the rest of our lives. We had gotten bicycles for transportation after arriving in Illinois, and I started thinking that it might be quite an educational adventure to ride our bikes back to California. Friends of ours were moving to Colorado, and when they heard of our plans they invited us to ride with them and share the driving as far as Colorado. We could start out on bicycles from there.

THE ADVENTURE BEGINS

It was the summer of 1976 when Andy and Cindy and I pedaled away from our friends' new home. Our dog, L'il Bit, was in a specially built basket on the front of Andy's bike, and the three of us were loaded with gear packed into saddlebags that fit over the rear fenders of our bicycles. We had hardly begun when the rain started. L'il Bit was the only one who stayed dry, her nose occasionally poking out from the covered basket as she looked around with curiosity before retreating to her dry bed. The rest of us donned our rain gear and braved the storms.

It was a year of flooding in Colorado. As we drove along in the steady rain, I nervously watched my eleven-year-old daughter in front of me as she braved the steep, slippery roads. We finally reached flat farmlands, with roads stretching out endlessly in front of us. We still had several miles left to go in the pouring rain one day when a flatbed truck passed by and then stopped. A man stepped out and shouted, "What in the world are you doing way out here?" We told him we were headed for the campground a few miles up the road and, shaking his head, he said, "Pile those bikes onto the back and get in. I'll drop you off." We gratefully accepted his offer.

Luck was with us when we found that the campground had a laundromat. After pitching our tent we were able to dry our things and crawl into toasty-warm sleeping bags. We set our little camp stove outside the flap of the tent and cooked spaghetti. For dessert we had dried pineapple. It was one of the most delicious meals I've ever had—and a memorable birthday. I turned twenty-nine that day.

By morning we had decided that there might be another way to enjoy this adventure home—after all, the trip was meant to be educational and fun. We decided to buy an old car and strap our bikes on top. Then we could drive the same schedule of miles we had planned to cover on bicycle, but now when we reached our destination for the day we could take our bikes down and explore the area. We found the perfect car. It was an old brown station wagon for five hundred dollars. Cindy decided to name it Randy—a premonition, we now laugh about, of the name of her future husband. Bikes tied on top, we started out again.

We drove through Indian reservations, learned to make necklaces out of seeds, stuck our noses into the crevices of pine trees to smell the sweet butterscotch-like scent, and fell in love with the Grand Canyon. We explored the surrounding area while we waited two weeks to get a reservation for an overnight hike to the bottom of the canyon. The timing was perfect, corresponding with Cindy's twelfth birthday.

Andy and Cindy started down together to spend the night at the bottom while I stayed in the campground with L'il Bit. In the morning I left the dog with fellow campers for the day and started out at daybreak to meet Andy and Cindy and hike back with them. Going down was a breeze. In order to get as far as possible I jogged most of the way. I was exhilarated when I passed the halfway mark. When Andy and Cindy came into sight, I was two-thirds of the way down.

It was a beautiful day and we were all in good spirits—for a while. As the sun and the temperature rose, Cindy's steps slowed to a drag. My attention was so focused on her that I was only mildly aware of my own protesting muscles. Andy, strong by nature and invigorated from his night in the canyon, went ahead to take care of L'il Bit and to get a campfire going for dinner.

Thank God for our angel that day. He was a friendly young hiker in his teens who stopped frequently to admire the scenery. We would pass him, then he would overtake us, then we would come upon him again, peering through the lens of his camera. Every time we passed he would grin at Cindy and cheer her on. Grumbling, and not yet appreciative of this grand experience, Cindy noticeably perked up whenever the young man came into view. His attention gave her the boost of adrenaline she needed to keep going. With much jubilation, we finally made it to the top.

After dinner I picked up our camp dishes to take them to a nearby sink, but my legs gave out from underneath me. I hit the ground with such force that I couldn't get up or walk on my own. My muscles were exhausted, and my legs were now bruised from thigh to knee. For several days I couldn't walk without leaning on Andy for support.

As we continued our drive south we reveled in the unique beauty of the desert and ended up in Tempe, Arizona, where we stayed for several months. Cindy was enrolled in school, and Andy and I attended college together after work. Evening was the only time it wasn't scorching hot. We bought a motorcycle and after classes I would climb on behind Andy and feel the cooling breeze against my face. The balmy nights of Arizona were magical.

It took us more than a year to get to California. Home, this time, was the Kent Motel in Lake Tahoe, which my parents had recently purchased with my youngest brother, Jim, and his wife. It had thirty-two rooms and ten apartments. My middle brother, Tim, lived in one of the apartments, Cindy and Andy and I moved into another, Jim and Lisa lived in the office quarters, and Dad and Mom drove up on the weekends. Mike and Emily, my older brother and his wife, ran the Sleepy Hollow motel down the street with Emily's parents.

Between both places we had plenty of catastrophes—pipes froze in the cold winters, toilets plugged up, rooms got damaged. One beautiful spring day we all gathered at the Kent to top off a pine tree in the courtyard that had become dangerously top-heavy. Just as the final cut was made, a blast of wind from out of nowhere snapped the bracing rope and whipped the severed section in the opposite direction. Fortunately all the rooms were empty when the projectile launched into the roof and lodged itself like an upside-down Christmas tree in the ceiling of a second-floor room.

Together we celebrated the births of two babies, a son born to Mike and Emily, and a daughter to Jim and Lisa a few months later. The days were busy, full of the fun and camaraderie and hard work of running a family business. And whenever time permitted, it was possible to escape into the vastly abundant and majestic forests and lakes that surrounded the town.

PEACE'S PATH CONVERGES WITH OURS

While Cindy and Andy and I had been slowly making our way across the country by car, Peace had been walking. We kept in touch by letter. She used a post office box in New Jersey where she told us a friend (who turned out to be her sister) picked up her mail and forwarded it each week. I was excited to see her again when she reached California. I invited my parents to a little church where she would be speaking in a nearby town. I had no idea how they would respond to Peace Pilgrim's unusual appearance, but they accepted the invitation and drove with us to the town of Pittsburg.

Rows of chairs were arranged in semicircles around the center where Peace stood, her smiling face radiant as she spoke in her usual dynamic style. She told the audience that her calling was to be a pilgrim, walking until humanity attained the spiritual awakening necessary to embrace the way of peace. She had said the same thing hundreds of times, and yet each time it sounded as fresh as if she were just discovering it.

The philosophy of the way of war, which all major nations still follow, she explained, is to accept that the end justifies the means. The way of war believes that violence can be overcome with more violence. The way of peace holds the perspective that the means determines the end. It is the philosophy that only good can overcome evil, that it takes love to overcome hate.

Peace told many stories of encounters she'd had during her years of walking, insisting that they were based on spiritual laws that worked for everyone, not just her. Early in her pilgrimage, for instance, when she crossed the desert for the first time, she told how she'd been walking late one night to keep warm. Somewhere in the middle of nowhere she walked by a car that was parked along the side of the road; a man called out, asking if she wanted to get in and warm up. She told him she didn't accept rides, but he said he was just parked for the night, so she got in.

He was a rough-looking individual, but she wasn't afraid. They talked for a while, and then he asked if she'd like to get a little sleep while she was there in the warm car. She said yes and curled right up and went to sleep.

When she woke up some time later he was sitting there looking puzzled. They talked for a time before he admitted to her that he'd meant her no good when she got in the car. "But you know," he said, "when you curled up so trustingly and went to sleep, I just couldn't touch you."

"Of course he couldn't," Peace commented, "because the good within him prevented him, even though he was surprised to find there was any good there. There are no accidents in the divine Plan, nor does God leave us unattended." When she walked away she looked back and saw him standing beside the car looking up at the stars. "I wondered if he might be thinking about God."

Peace Pilgrim told another story about a time when she was hit by a disturbed teenage boy. The anecdote illustrates, as she put it, "an obedient attitude toward God's law of love even under very difficult circumstances." She wanted to help this boy do something that he really wanted to do in order to bring something good into his life. She knew he was violent at times. He'd once attacked a group of people with a hatchet; he'd even beaten his own mother so badly that she was hospitalized for a couple of weeks. Yet, another time he had lovingly nursed her through an illness.

He was a tall young man, six foot three, and built like a football player. When Peace inquired about what he'd really like to do, he talked about taking a walking trip into the hills. He was afraid to go alone because he thought he might break a leg or something and be left there helpless. But he couldn't find anyone to go with him because everyone was afraid of him. Peace said she'd go.

They started out on a good note, but when they were up on a hill-top a thundershower suddenly came up. Terrified, he went off the beam. He hurled himself toward Peace, his eyes wild, hitting at her as he came. He had a large pack on his back, and in his imbalanced state he was as clumsy as a drunken man. Peace could have run, but instead she raised her arms to ward off his blows and stood looking at him. "I saw the good in him and I reached for it. I prayed for him. I felt the deepest compassion for this young man who was sick enough to hit an old woman. The hitting stopped very quickly. He was bewildered by this new situation because never before had his hatred been met with love." The boy said, "You didn't hit back. My mother always hits back."

Then he was struck by remorse. For quite some time he was overcome by self-condemnation, and then he went limp, the fight in him gone. "I guess you're going home now," he said to Peace, "and I don't blame you." She said, "No, I'm not going to leave you. But the next time, perhaps you'll think before you harm anyone."

Peace Pilgrim concluded that some people might consider her method to have failed since he had hit her. "But looking back over a period of years I can only say, did my method fail? Did God's method of love fail? What are a few bruises on my body in comparison to the transformation of a human life? He was never violent again. He is a useful citizen today. Of course God's laws work—when we use them."

The stories Peace told happened early on in her pilgrimage; she called them her tests. In another one she was staying with a family on a farm. The parents had to go into town on an errand, and the daughter, a young girl, didn't want to go. Peace, who was on the front porch answering her mail, said she would watch the child. At some point she looked up and saw a man chasing the terrified girl into the barn. Peace ran after them. When she entered the barn she saw the girl cowering in fright in a corner, the man advancing toward her slowly and deliberately. "Of course you attract to you the very thing that you fear, and I knew the girl was in great danger." Peace moved in front of the man, placing herself between him and the girl.

> I have never felt such power in my body as when I stood and looked at that poor psychologically sick man with loving compassion. He stopped in his tracks, almost as though he had hit something. When you do God's will, you receive God's protection. He looked at me for quite a while, then he turned and walked away.
>
> Don't ever underestimate the power of the way of love. It reaches the good in the other fellow and is disarming. And it can be used in small things, where nobody's life is in danger. Just little things. And it works not only between individuals, but on a collective level, between nations, if nations had the courage to use them.

Peace's stories were like the tales of a traveling angel who saw and found the good in people. I had my doubts about whether or not such trust would work for the average individual, let alone a whole nation, but I wanted to think it was possible.

At the end of Peace's presentation several people, including my parents, gathered around her, eager to ask questions. In talking about her solitary pilgrimage, Peace mentioned that friends had been urging her for years to lead a retreat so that she could spend more time with them. She had decided to give it a try and was planning two inspirational and educational retreats—one in Alaska and one in Hawaii. "How do we join up?" my parents asked eagerly, and in the next moment we were all signed up for the first trip.

11

Land of Vastness

*Genuine beginnings begin within us, even when they
are brought to our attention by external opportunities.*

WILLIAM BRIDGES

In July of 1979, eighteen of us rendezvoused at the airport in Seattle
to begin a ten-day experience of living simply. We had been asked to
bring only one set of clothes, dressing in layers—bathing suit, shorts,
long pants, jacket, and so on. We were to carry a sleeping bag and a
small carry-on bag with essentials. I don't think anyone traveled as
lightly as Peace suggested, but most of us had pared down substan-
tially from what we were used to traveling or camping with.

Andy and I arrived the night before our early-morning flight, prepared to sleep in the waiting area as Peace had suggested. A few people in the group opted for a nearby motel room while others, like us,
were eager to get right into the adventure of living like Peace. Peace
herself arrived just before midnight in the company of two elderly
white-haired women. I woke up briefly, smiling to myself at the idea of
being asleep on the floor of an airport terminal, waiting to go to Alaska
with a room full of strangers who all seemed to be well into their
mature years. I drifted back to sleep until five-thirty, when everyone
started getting up and gathering gear together to meet the plane.

As we stood in line I noticed a man with a salt-and-pepper beard
and warm brown eyes whom I hadn't noticed the night before. He was

leaning against the wall across the room, talking to my father. At first I thought he was a priest, but I saw he wore the same casual clothes as the rest of us. When we were introduced on the plane, I found out that his name was also Andy. To avoid confusing him with my husband, we gave him the nickname A. Z. Although a dozen years older than Andy and me, he was the next youngest person after us. This wasn't the college-aged crowd I was expecting.

It was a three-hour flight. Peace organized us by passing out slips of paper with the numbers one, two, or three on them. It became a ritual I looked forward to each day. The number indicated whether we would be riding in car number one, two, or three. Andy was driver number one, in charge of car number one. A. Z. was driver number two, and Archie, my father, was driver number three. Peace herself rotated each day among the three cars.

As the plane descended into Anchorage, we were greeted with a breathtaking view of sparkling water and rugged snowcapped mountain peaks. We checked out our rental cars and divided into groups according to our numbers. It was an effective way to separate people who had come together and, over the ten days we had together, helped all of us to get better acquainted. I loved drawing the car Peace was riding in so I could hear her stories. Six of us would crowd into each of the three cars with our bags and gear and head off for the day.

The trip was designed to give us an experience of living simply and included eating a vegetarian fare, taking most of our meals and sleeping outdoors. Knowing my penchant for eating healthy vegetarian food, Peace gave me the job of standing at the check-out stands when we did our group shopping, so I could read labels and make sure we were getting wholesome, nutritious food. A. Z. took it upon himself to be my tester, doing his best to distract me long enough to get some contraband substance past me. He would roll his eyes innocently and Peace would laugh with the rest of the group when I would discover a pack of Hostess Twinkies before they got to the cashier.

From Anchorage, where beautiful baskets of colorful flowers hung everywhere, we headed into the vast wilderness toward

Fairbanks. Sleeping outdoors under the Alaskan summer skies was an experience in itself. At 11 P.M. we would have to shield our eyes from the sun and, if still awake, we could watch the sun set at midnight. For three hours we would lie in the twilight, under a vast, luminous sky devoid of stars. Sunrise came just after 3 A.M. and by the time I roused myself a couple of hours later Peace would be up attending to a camp-fire. With the short nights and extra sunlight I felt refreshed and full of energy with much less sleep than usual.

Peace had told us to bring light bedding for moderate summer weather, but I shivered in my sleeping bag in the cool evenings. Peace was sleeping in one of the cars, I imagined for some privacy, since she was well-adjusted to living out-of-doors. My parents slept in the car Archie was in charge of, and two elderly sisters slept in the third. After a few nights of shivering on the ground, I decided to try out the open trunk of one of the cars and discovered that Andy and I could fit comfortably enough and keep cozy and warm.

Our first picnic was in a forest carpeted with a myriad of wildflowers. With hearty appetites we relished what was to become our staple lunch, peanut butter sandwiches. It was estimated at the end of our ten days together that we had each consumed a full pound of peanut butter. Most of the greens for our salads came from the University at Fairbanks, where we volunteered, in exchange, to weed the garden of lamb's-quarters.

Between intermittent rains and downpours we toured Fairbanks and the University, where some of us accompanied Peace to a talk she gave to a Sociology class. I arrived early and sat in back where I could watch the reaction of the students to Peace. Many were slouched in their seats and snickered when she entered, greeting them with a booming, "What a joy to be here!" Before long the same students were leaning forward, completely engrossed in her talk.

Alaska was a grand adventure. We took a paddleboat down the Chena River. We drove miles into the wilderness to Chena Hot Springs, which was not yet completed and where mosquitoes really are the size of butterflies. We took a bus ride through Mount McKinley

National Park, now called Denali; there, ptarmigans in their brown summer plumage waddled across the road, we had to swerve to avoid a lynx, and a golden eagle soared overhead. And we took a twenty-minute ski lift to the top of Mount Alyeska, where we climbed higher still to stand on glaciers.

SPIRIT OF THE LAW

Living outdoors and traveling in crowded cars was hard on some. One or two people left the trip early on, and for others it remained difficult and tiring at times. Tempers occasionally flared.

Once, we were in a beautiful state park toward the end of a day when the group started to question Peace about where we would spend the night. Peace pointed to a small hill a short distance away and indicated the meadow on the other side. "But there's no camping in this park," one of the men informed her. "Oh, we're not going to camp," she replied. "We won't have a fire or anything. We're just going to sleep."

Shortly after that the same man came back and said, "Peace, I just talked to the park ranger and asked if we could sleep here. He said we're not allowed to stay overnight." We all looked at Peace.

"Never ask!" she scolded him gently. "If you ask, authorities are in a position of having to enforce the letter of the law. I live by the spirit of the law, always respecting where I am and leaving it better than I found it. Now that you've asked we'll have to leave."

Though the sun was still up, the hour was late. We had to pile into the cars and drive many miles before we could find a place to pull over and sleep. The debate was hot in my car. "How could she do that! Expecting us to break the law!" I sat silently, quietly relishing the words Peace had spoken: *spirit of the law*. The phrase washed over me like a refreshing shower.

We traveled fifteen hundred miles throughout central Alaska. Amid the vast and rugged beauty, what stands out most in my mind is the small and animated figure of Peace Pilgrim giving morning and evening talks around the campfire, sharing her own spiritual awakening and what she called her steps toward inner peace. "There is no glimpse of the light without walking the path. You can't get it from anyone else, nor can you give it to anyone. You take whatever steps seem easiest for you, and as you take a few steps it will be easier to take a few more."

PEACE'S STEPS TOWARD INNER PEACE

Peace divided the steps she had taken in her own life into three categories: Preparations, Purifications, and Relinquishments.

Preparations

The first preparation, Peace explained, has to do with a right attitude toward life.

> There was a time when I was a surface liver who stayed right in the froth on the surface. There are millions of escapists. There are millions of surface livers. They never find anything really worthwhile because you must delve very deeply for life's verities and realities. There was a time when, if I was confronted with a problem, I tried to get rid of it. I tried to get somebody else to solve it for me. But then I began to realize that every problem that came to me I was capable of solving if I turned to God for help.

Problems, she pointed out, serve a purpose. Every time we solve a problem according to the highest light we have, we attain a little more spiritual growth. The bigger the problem, the greater the opportunity for personal growth.

> I began to face my problems with anticipation. Here's a problem—what can I learn from this? And I began to work meaningfully to solve those problems. And I also began to realize that I had a part to play in solving the great collective problems that

are set before all of us. Problems like attaining world peace. I began to pray about those problems and as I prayed about them I was motivated to act upon them because right prayer motivates to right action. Through solving personal problems and helping to solve collective problems, I grew and grew. So I wouldn't wish for people a life without problems. I would wish for them the strength to meaningfully solve their problems and attain spiritual growth.

The second preparation has to do with living in harmony with God's laws, which are the same for everyone. These are the principles that govern the universe and run through religious teachings. They can be studied alone or in a group, but they have to be lived out individually. The same cause-and-effect applies to spiritual and physical laws alike, but we have free will as to whether or not we follow spiritual law. When we do, we experience an inner harmony and peace. When we don't, we create difficulties for ourselves. Peace explained it in this way:

> If you're out of harmony through ignorance, you suffer somewhat. If you know better and are still out of harmony, you suffer a lot. You actually make things worse for yourself if you know and do not do. Let me give you an example of this. I asked two men the same question. They were both coughing their heads off and smoking one cigarette after another and I said to them, "Do you think perhaps it would ease your throat a little if you would stop smoking for a while?" The first was a big burly man who did heavy work and he said, "Why I always smoke when I have a cold. You know it kills disease germs." He will suffer physically. The second was a college professor and he said, "I know this thing is bad for me in every way," and kept right on smoking. He will suffer not only physically but spiritually, because he knows and does not do.

The third preparation is unique for every person and has to do with finding one's individual part in the overall scheme of things. Everyone comes into this life with a special job to do, with his or her own unique place in life. Peace began her search by taking time each day, maybe an hour, to walk alone in the beauty of nature. She called this walking meditation a time of receptive silence and found that wonderful insights sometimes came then. When they did she would put them into practice.

"I realize that in most lives it isn't one big thing," Peace told us, "but many little things. And I also realize that most people are not called to do some unusual job but a well-recognized, useful task in society. You can begin by doing the good things you feel motivated toward, even if they are small things at first. You give these priority in your life over all the superficial things that customarily clutter human lives."

The last of the preparations is to simplify life, to bring inner and outer well-being into harmony. "Unnecessary possessions are unnecessary burdens. If you have them, you have to take care of them." Need levels are different for everyone, Peace realized, and very few people could live comfortably at the basic level she had chosen for herself. Families require the stability of a family center, for instance, and needs go beyond physical needs. The things we don't need but hold on to are the things that become burdens.

Peace offered a story to illustrate this concept.

I knew a dear lady who was up in her years, and I was concerned because she was working much too hard. And I said to her, "Do you really need to work so hard? You have only yourself to support." And she said, "Well you see, I have to pay rent on a five-room house." "A five-room house?" I said to her. "But you're alone in the world. Couldn't you live happily in one room?" "Oh yes," she said sadly, "but I have furniture for a five-room house." And this woman was actually working her fingers to the bone to provide a proper home for that furniture!

Living a simple lifestyle, Peace found, can bring a sense of freedom and harmony into life. This is true not only for individuals, but also for society as a whole. There is a great disparity between people who have so much more than they need and people who don't have enough. The value our culture has given to the material side has pulled the world out of harmony to such a degree that our inner well-being lags behind our outer well-being.

"It's because," Peace elaborated, "as a world we have gotten ourselves so far out of harmony, so way off on the material side, that when we discover something like nuclear energy, we are still capable of putting it into a bomb and using it to kill people. The valid research for the future is on the inner side, on the psychological side, so that we will be able to bring these two into balance; so that we will know how to use well the outer well-being we already have."

Purifications

Then Peace discovered that certain purifications were required of her. The first she called purification of the body, having to do with sensible living habits—eating right and getting plenty of rest, fresh air, sunshine, and contact with nature. The body can be considered the temple of the spirit and should be treated with the kind of respect one would have for a temple. Peace also thought of her body as her clay garment. "If you only had one suit of clothes, you'd take good care of it."

We wouldn't think of getting the best use out of an automobile by putting in inferior gas or neglecting to change the oil or keep it tuned up. The same principles work with regard to the body. "You'd think this might be the first area in which people would be willing to work," said Peace, "but from practical experience I've discovered it's often the last, because it might mean getting rid of some of our bad habits—and there is nothing that we cling to more tenaciously!"

The second purification is the purification of thought. "Your thoughts are so powerful that if you had any idea of their power you would never think a negative thought." Conversely, positive thoughts are a powerful influence for good. Peace focused her thoughts on the best thing that could happen in a given situation, including world events.

Whenever we hear negative predictions of disaster, for example, Peace advised putting our thoughts in the opposite direction, toward the best possible outcome. The only thing that can ever be predicted, she said, is the trend in things. "You can never say what the outcome will be, because we are constantly able to turn that prediction in another direction—in a positive direction—if we get together on that."

When thoughts are charged with negative ideas and feelings, they can also make us sick, as doctors and scientists now recognize. Peace was aware of the connection between the mind and body long before *psychoneuroimmunology* was a recognized word. She spoke about several people she had worked with, including a sixty-five-year-old man with a chronic illness. She recognized that he had some bitterness in him, but she couldn't put her finger on it at first. He was well respected in his community and got along well with his wife and grown children. But as Peace probed she discovered he was harboring bitterness against his father, who had been dead for many years.

The father had sent the man's brother to college but not him. Even though the man had done well financially, he resented the fact that he'd never gotten to go to college. As Peace spoke with him he began to realize that at the time he'd left home, there were still two other children remaining. After the sister left, only the youngest son remained and the father could afford to send him to college. When the man realized that his father had done the best he could, he was able to let go of his bitterness; the chronic illness began to fade away until it was gone.

"If you're harboring the slightest bitterness toward anyone," Peace taught, "or any unkind thoughts of any sort whatever, you must get rid of them quickly. They aren't hurting anyone but you. It isn't enough to say and do right things, you must also think right things before your life can come into harmony."

The last purifications has to do with desires and motives. When thoughts are focused on superficial desires of the self-centered nature, the God-centered nature lies dormant, waiting to be called on. Peace discovered that happiness and joy come when we find and do our part in life by awakening the higher nature within.

"Your motive, if you are to find inner peace, must be outgoing—it must be service. It must be giving, not getting." Peace told us about an architect she'd met who had worked himself into an illness. He was good at his job and it was obviously his right work, she said, but his motive was to make a lot of money. Before she left town she talked to him about the joy of service, telling him that once he experienced it he wouldn't want to go back to self-centered living. Three years later she walked into his town again, and he was so radiant she hardly recognized him. He was still an architect but now he was excited about helping the people he made plans for. "You see," he told her, "I'm designing it this way to fit into their budget, and then I'll set it on their plot of land like this to make it look nice. . . ." His business had increased tremendously, his wife told Peace, and people were coming from miles around for his house plans.

"I've met a few people who had to change their jobs in order to change their lives," said Peace, "but I've met many more people who merely had to change their motive to service in order to change their lives."

Relinquishments

The final category Peace outlined has to do with relinquishments—relinquishing self-will, feelings of separateness, and attachments. Self-will is that part of us that is sometimes motivated to do or say something mean. Once we have relinquished self-will, Peace taught, we have found inner peace. It's as though we have two selves or two natures—a lower one that governs selfishly, and a higher one that "stands ready to use you gloriously." The lower nature might be motivated to do or say something mean. We can refrain from doing an unkind thing, Peace said, not by suppressing it, but by using the energy to do or say something good instead. She recounted this story to illustrate the point:

I knew a woman who played the piano. She had a quick temper and a sharp tongue, and every once in a while she would be motivated to say something hurtful to her husband or one of her teenage children, and her household was in a constant uproar. She got the idea of taking it out on the piano, and after that when her family came home and found her playing the piano in the midst of preparing dinner they left her alone. They knew there was a reason for it. I know another woman who scrubs floors and a man who gets out the manual lawn mower and mows the lawn. You can use the energy that comes to do something constructive.

The next relinquishment is the feeling of separateness. We start out as children, Peace explained, feeling ourselves to be separate and judging everything from the perspective of seeing ourselves as the center of the universe. Even when we grow up and know better intellectually, we often still see the world from that perspective.

"In reality we are all cells in the same body of humanity," said Peace. "Every cell is of equal value and worth. When you know that, you know what it is to love your neighbor as yourself. You know your neighbor is just as important as you are—no more and no less. You know that anything that hurts anybody, anywhere, really hurts all of us."

When we work for our own interests, Peace went on, we are just one cell working against all those other cells. We're way out of harmony. But when we begin to work for the good of the whole, we find ourselves in harmony with the people around us. "It's the easy, harmonious way to live."

The next relinquishment is that of attachments. Material things are here to be used, but we need to be able to relinquish them when we no longer need them. Peace explained it in this way:

Anything that you can't relinquish when it has outlived its usefulness possesses you. And in this material age a great many of us are possessed by our possessions. We are bound, we are tied, we are not free.

There is another kind of possession. You do not possess any other human being, no matter how closely related that other person may be. No husband owns his wife. No wife owns her husband. No parents own their children. When we think we possess them we try to run their lives for them, which develops into an extremely disharmonious situation.

It is only when we realize that we don't own the people who are close to us, Peace taught, that we are able to let them live according to their own inner guidance, and we stop trying to run their lives. And then we find that we can live in harmony with one another.

The final relinquishment Peace spoke of was the relinquishment of negative feelings:

> I want to mention one negative feeling which the nicest people still experience, and that is worry. Worry is not concern, which motivates you to do everything possible in a situation. Worry is a useless mulling over of things we cannot change. If you worry, you agonize over the past which you should have forgotten long ago, or you're apprehensive over the future which hasn't even come yet. We tend to skim right over the present. Since this is the only moment that one can live, if you don't live it, you never really get around to living at all. If you do live this present moment, you tend not to worry.

For ten days in Alaska we explored the beautiful land by day and listened to Peace's inspiring talks before going to sleep at night. In the morning I would wake up anxious to get started and not miss a moment. One early morning I left Peace at the campfire to go to the bathroom near the edge of the campground. When I got there the entrance to the bathroom was blocked by a pack of wild dogs, who emitted low growls as the hair on their backs stood up. I backed away and returned to the security of the group.

Peace saw me coming and said, "That was quick!" I told her about the dogs. "Don't be afraid," she told me. "The dogs won't challenge you when they know that you're the master, not them." She beckoned me to follow and walked toward the bathroom with firm steps. When we got there (me following respectfully behind) Peace looked at the dogs and pointed into the surrounding woods. "Go on," she commanded. "Be gone now!" and the dogs obediently got up, tails between their legs, and trotted off.

The two Andys and I relished every opportunity to be with Peace Pilgrim, and she began to refer to us affectionately as the Three Musketeers. On one afternoon when the rest of the group had gone to a restaurant in Anchorage, we lingered on the green grass of a park, happy with peanut butter sandwiches and a quiet interlude with Peace. It was the first of many such moments shared among the four of us over the next few years.

On this day she spoke to us about the natural unfolding of insight or intuition; this development is a part of the spiritual growth process. Sometimes, she said, she would look at a person and his or her face would seem to ripple, as a pond ripples when a pebble is tossed in. Then when the ripples cleared she would see the person as he or she had been in a recent or significant life. Laughing, she looked at A. Z. "Like right now," she said, "I see you as a monk or priest." I had already told A. Z. about my first impression of him, and we all burst out laughing. Peace cautioned us:

> I don't think we should ever make a big fuss out of this phenomenon, but it does happen. Finding lost objects, knowing what people are thinking, seeing auras, seeing past lives—as you go on you're going to have an inkling of these things. It's natural, but it should never be forced. I always think about the bud of a flower. If you give it proper conditions, it will open into a beautiful flower, but if you are impatient and try to tear the petals open, you permanently injure the flower. The flower can be equated with a human life. Give the spiritual growing-up the proper growing conditions, and it will open into a thing of beauty.

We went to a museum on the last day and had lunch on the grounds before going to the airport. A tiny woman came out of the museum and, looking around, spotted Peace on the grass. Walking over to her, she said, "I'm waiting for my bus and I feel safe here by you." Her characteristic Eskimo face was creased with wrinkles and she looked out from smiling eyes. For almost an hour she regaled us with stories of her native life and when she left, it was time for us to leave too. All too soon the adventure had come to an end. We said good-bye to this land of vastness.

12

Sojourn in Paradise

The real voyage of discovery consists not in seeking
new landscapes but in having new eyes.

MARCEL PROUST

It was the summer of 1980 and my first trip to Hawaii. I was with
Peace Pilgrim and sixteen others on another inspirational and educational retreat. This time Andy wasn't able to come; Cindy stayed with
him and then joined me on Oahu at the end of the retreat. The smell
and feel of the tropics hit me the moment I stepped off the plane. The
intoxicating fragrance of gardenias and plumeria hung in the mois-
ture-laden air. For the next three weeks my spirits soared and my feet
barely touched the ground.

Once again, this was to be an experience of living simply, sleeping outdoors, fixing vegetarian meals over an open fire, and enjoying the beauty of nature. We expected to travel in three cars, but
because of an error in rental car reservations, only two station wag-
ons were available to us. Four of us, including A. Z., had been with
the Alaska group the previous year; this time A. Z. was promoted to
driver number one, with a new recruit, Richard, as driver number
two. We drove off with nine people in each car. Luggage was piled
on the roof, under our feet, and behind the rear seats. Along with a
woman named Jean, I squeezed into the area behind the seats in car
number one, happily tucked in with sleeping bags and suitcases. I

could have been strapped on the roof and it wouldn't have dampened my enthusiasm.

We landed on the Big Island and flew on short flights to Kauai, Maui, and Oahu. The islands blur together between my memories of flowers, scented air, sandy beaches, volcanoes, and nights spent staring up into star-filled skies. It happened that my thirty-third birthday fell on a day when we were camped on a high mountain where, in spite of our being in Hawaii, we were quite chilly.

I woke up in the predawn hours and decided I'd treat myself to a shower even though there was no hot water in the campground. When I got to the bathroom, I was surprised to find that someone was in the shower ahead of me. I waited several minutes, listening to a swishing sound. After a time I cleared my throat, and Peace's head popped out.

"Good morning!" she greeted me cheerfully. "I'll be right out." In a moment she walked out wet from head to foot, having put back on the clothes she had been swishing clean while taking a shower. The shower water was so cold that I jumped out as quickly as I had gotten in—and here was Peace smiling, soaking in it!

The day started, as most did, with all of us gathered around a campfire sipping tea and having breakfast, listening to Peace as she answered questions and told stories. After breakfast we drove along the coast looking at the brilliant blue of the Pacific Ocean on one side and lush forests on the other, where nearly all the native flowering plants and forest birds are endemic, being found in Hawaii and nowhere else.

We stopped briefly at a remote Buddhist temple. There, we met an orange-robed monk from Tibet. He was wearing a paper hat for protection from the sun and scraping paint off some old boards, no doubt with the intention of reusing them. His gentle face looked timeless.

From there we drove to Volcano National Park and walked through a forest of tree ferns to of one of the world's most active volcanoes, Halema'uma'u. We made our way down the Chain of Craters Road, stopping to explore along the way.

At a bird sanctuary we got out and walked among some of the world's rarest plants. In few other forests can one see so many different kinds of trees growing in so small an area. At the end of the trail we found a giant koa tree. It was probably hundreds of years old, but because the nearly uniform climate prevents the development of annual growth rings, it was difficult to tell. One heavy branch had pulled away and broken off, leaving the core of the tree open and vulnerable. It was an awesome sight.

Later we hiked a path to a lava tube, a tunnel formed in the lava as it cooled. Moisture dripped from the ceiling, and we had to step around large puddles. Dim lanterns along the sides cast a soft light on the eerie beauty as we made our way through. As I gazed into the stars that night, I imagined that all the spectacular sights we had seen that day were special gifts, sent to me from the universe for my birthday.

On the island of Maui a few days later, we traversed the winding road that led to the Seven Sacred Falls, taking a detour to visit the quiet little church where Charles Lindbergh was buried. When we arrived at the falls, we found clear blue pools at the bottom of each tier, the last one running out into the ocean. We bathed in the pools, swam, washed our hair, and basked in the sun. It was as breathtaking as any paradise I could imagine.

That evening we made camp on a plateau above the falls, in a downpour that lasted much of the night. By morning the rain had stopped, and as the sun's early rays touched the wet landscape it was transformed into a sparkling fairyland.

DIVINE PROTECTION

Several days later while we were making camp on a sandy beach, a policeman came by. Although we had a camping permit, he told us it was a dangerous place because someone had been killed there. "Don't worry about us," Peace told him. "We'll be fine." Although most of us felt very comfortable staying on the beach, when we gathered around the campfire that night a member of the group chided

Peace for putting us in danger. Peace said she was concerned about all the fear that was being perpetuated on these beautiful islands:

> A certain amount of being sensible is good, such as looking up and down a street before you cross. But I don't believe any amount of fear is healthy. I believe we are required to do everything possible for ourselves and therefore when I walk out onto a street I always look both ways. If you're going to be fearful—let's say about sleeping on a beach—you must be terrified every time you sleep in your own home. Look how many people are killed in their own home. Or when you sleep in a hotel room. Look how many people are killed in hotel rooms. This can lead to ridiculous behavior.

Peace went on to talk about what she called divine protection. "We all have protection, or guardians. And the more a life is spent in service, the greater the protection and number of guardians."

Then she told stories about times when she had felt unsafe while riding in cars. The first time she was picked up by a man who had been drinking. She was carrying a driver's license at the time and offered to drive but he declined, so she got out of the car. She was picked up a few minutes later by someone else and had gone only a short distance when she spotted the car she had been in earlier. It had gone off the road and sideswiped a tree—breaking the glass and caving in the roof on the passenger side. The driver was cut but not badly hurt.

Another time she was with a man who was driving recklessly, and she got out because she felt it was unsafe; that time she never saw the driver again. On another occasion she was in a car with two high school students who were racing down a stretch of highway called The Grapevine near Los Angeles, "seeing how fast they could get the old Chevy to go," but that time she felt safe and stayed in the car.

"I do have a sense of complete protection," Peace told us. "If I felt the slightest apprehension about being here, I would take the whole crowd off the beach. So I think we should not be apprehensive. I don't think apprehension can do anything except attract. 'That which I feared came upon me.'"

KARMA

The only thing we are not protected against, Peace taught, is our own karma or carelessness—karma being the law of cause-and-effect, "as you sow so shall you reap," as seen over the span of many lifetimes.

"There are physical laws, like gravity, that have to be obeyed. You would never get to the ground safely without a parachute if you stepped out of a tenth-story window. And physical laws apply to the food we eat. But there are also the spiritual laws of love and harmony. Those who get ulcers as a result of hating someone prove to themselves, if they have the eyes to see, that the law of karma works. As it is said, hate injures the hater, not the hated. And debts can be carried over from a previous life."

While discussing karma Peace told us about a soldier who had come to her, asking if there was anything he could do to make up for the killing he had participated in.

"The best way to rid yourself of all bad karma," she counseled, "is to get busy serving in any way you can. When you have given enough, you will know God and find inner peace—for it is in giving that we receive."

Service, she believed, is a better way than paying in kind for our mistakes; it is also the way to inner peace. Peace advised the soldier to spend his life working for peace. He followed her advice and joined a peace organization, eventually becoming one of its leaders.

"The universe is always forgiving—but we don't always forgive ourselves, and guilt can cast a lingering shadow. You can use the same energy you've been using to condemn yourself to improve yourself."

The Earth life, Peace said, is a drop in eternity, an excursion we make many times on our journey toward wholeness and inner peace. We always have free will, and every problem that comes serves a purpose. From this point of view there is little room for being a victim.

Even the family into which we are born, she said, is a choice we make. We choose our family of origin in order to learn the lessons we need.

Peace described the soul, before entering the Earth life, as being given a choice of a half-dozen or so problems to choose from. A timid soul might take one and say, "That's enough for me!" and may appear to do well in life. A more courageous soul might say, "I'll take it all on. Give me all six!" This life may appear to be full of ups and downs but, if successful, can lead to six times the spiritual growth. Hence, Peace often said, we can recognize problems as opportunities in disguise.

TEACHERS AND GUARDIANS

Each night around the campfire, under tropical star-studded skies, Peace regaled us with her mystical perceptions:

> Everyone has both a teacher and a guide, or a guardian angel, as a guide is sometimes called. The guide is customarily available to you in your waking state. Not always with you necessarily, but any emergency would call your guide to help you. Your teacher is customarily with you at night in your sleep state. Besides that, you may have more than one teacher and more than one guide, and if you're doing some special work you may have a helper in that regard. A musician or an artist, for instance, may have a special helper.

It isn't good to try and get to know these teachers, because if you get to know them you bind yourself to them. At some point you could take a much higher teacher but you've bound yourself to the one you have. Just simply let this progression take place. You don't have to do anything about it. Just let them come and go as your need changes.

We spent our last night camping on a beautiful beach on Oahu. A. Z. and I led Peace to a moonlit cove of white sand, where we had laid out a sleeping bag for her earlier. We left to join the rest of the group and promised to wake her up at dawn. In the early morning light we entered the cove where Peace was still sleeping peacefully. Much to our surprise, a fully open yellow flower had sprouted next to her head. We woke her up, exclaiming our wonderment at the flower growing where there had been nothing but white sand the evening before. She jumped up, straightening her clothes, and stated matter-of-factly, "There's a logical explanation for everything."

Time had seemed suspended that summer in Hawaii. Leaving was like waking up from a beautiful dream. The trip had been a magical excursion, a time to suspend ideas of limitation and to travel in mystical realms.

13

Testing the Water

You must give if you want to receive. Let the center of your
being be one of giving, giving, giving. You can't give too much,
and you will discover you cannot give without receiving.

PEACE PILGRIM

Inspired by Peace and our own yearning to be of service, the two Andys and I departed for Port-au-Prince, the capital of Haiti, to work with Mother Teresa's Missionaries of Charity. We arrived at the airport François Duvalier and were immediately caught up in masses of people. As we drove into town, even the dry crusty earth reflected the poverty that was visible everywhere.

By the following day we had met with the head nun, Sister Carmeline, and toured the facilities—a combination dispensary and clinic, a children's home, and a home for the destitute and dying. We were to split our days mostly between the first two, helping out occasionally at the home for the dying.

The nuns, dressed in white saris with blue trim, were a striking community of cheerful acquiescence who, with loving devotion, followed the high ideals of Mother Teresa:

> If sometimes our poor people have had to die of starvation, it is not because God didn't care for them, but because you and I didn't give, were not instruments of love in the hands of God, to give

them that bread, to give them that clothing; because we did not recognize Him, when once more Christ came in distressing disguise—in the hungry man, in the homeless child, and seeking for shelter. Because we cannot see Christ we cannot express our love to Him; but our neighbors we can always see, and we can do for them what, if we saw Him, we would like to do for Christ.

POOREST OF THE POOR

The clinic stood downtown behind locked iron gates next to the Catholic church. On a typical morning the crowd would already be thick when we arrived a few minutes before eight. There would be an assortment of people with various ailments, perhaps a leper, mothers with small, malnourished babies, and others who came for tuberculosis shots and treatment.

The people who stood waiting for the gates to open were the poorest of the poor. It was surprising to see that some were dressed fairly well and were relatively clean. The decent clothes were due to a gesture of benevolence by the ruling family, in particular Michele Duvalier, wife of "Baby Doc," as her husband was nicknamed. Others arrived in the same rags week after week. How some managed to stay even superficially clean was a mystery, considering the lack of water for even the most basic hygiene.

Every morning long lines formed at various locations throughout the city where water spigots were turned on for a short period of time. People stood holding receptacles of all sizes—some as tiny as aspirin bottles—waiting their turn and hoping the water would run long enough for them to gather what they could for the day.

When we arrived, the crowd would part to let us through. The spontaneous reaction to white people, *blancs* as they called us, was one of simple respect. It was generally assumed that blancs were rich, privileged, and sometimes generous.

At the gate we would call out to Phillip John, gatekeeper in the morning and student when the clinic turned into a school in the afternoon. Those who attended school were the poor children of St. Joseph's parish. Phillip John was a handsome young teenager who often joined us in the morning, notebook and pen in hand, as we awaited the arrival of the nuns. He was enthusiastic and fun and loved teaching us French and Creole and learning English in return.

The first room on the right was used as a first-aid station where the bandaging and cleansing of wounds were tended to and shots were given. On the other side of the alley a table stretched across open double doors laden with various tablet and liquid medications, cleansers, and lotions. At the far end of the same room, school desks were pushed to the sides, and a dressing screen provided some privacy as we treated people for scabies. When there was an American doctor or dentist on hand, another room was set up for that person's use.

Time didn't have the same application in Haiti as it did in the United States. The nuns would arrive somewhere between eight-fifteen and nine o'clock. Before any activity started, we would stand behind the nuns in a little stock room and bow our heads with them as they intoned a special prayer: "Dear Lord, Thou Great Physician, I kneel before Thee, since every good and perfect gift must come from Thee. I pray, give skill to my hand, clear vision to my mind, kindness and sympathy to my heart. Give me singleness of purpose, strength to lift at least part of the burden of my suffering fellowmen, and true realization of the privilege that is mine. Take from my heart all guile and worldliness that with the simple faith of a child I may rely on Thee."

Once everything was prepared, someone at the gate would let people in a few at a time, directing them to the different areas. On Saturdays, which held TB clinics exclusively, a food line was set up. Participants were required to carry blue cards as a form of identification for the food program. Usually the fare was powdered milk and crackers or a soy protein powder.

Everywhere, we observed a lack of the most basic necessities for proper hygiene—and the clinic was no exception. In the first-aid section there was a row of old chairs and stools for the patients. The floor of rough cement was swept and sometimes mopped, but dust blew in from the barred windows and collected everywhere. Supply cabinets with mesh or cloth doors lined two walls. In the center of the room a long wooden table was wiped down and then set up with bandages, ointments, and equipment for injections. A small sterilizer was plugged in first thing, and all the needles and syringes were prepared for the day's use.

The first patients to enter would sit in a row of chairs; the line continued out the door and along the walls. We would then begin mass treatment of every imaginable affliction. Many conditions were visually shocking to incoming volunteers from the States, who at times were simply unable to cope with the enormity of suffering and affliction. Some had to leave. Others remained and were touched by the simple acceptance and resilience of those being treated.

The general clinic took place on Mondays, Wednesdays, and Fridays. Many came in for routine bandage changes. It was funny to watch a new volunteer attempt to help one of these regulars. Most were barefoot and illiterate. They would sit passively and smile angelically if you looked in their direction. Often they would burst into lengthy dissertations in Creole. No matter how much we interrupted them with, *"Mí pa pale Creole. Mí comprend petit"* ("I do not speak Creole. I understand little"), still they would continue, usually speaking louder and faster.

When attending to wounds, a strict adherence to procedure had to be followed. Otherwise a very stern expression would appear on the patient's face. His or her head would shake in disapproval. Newly arrived volunteers would look exasperated and puzzled as an equally puzzled Haitian would rapidly chatter, pointing to the table, settling for no less than the usual treatment. Patients were particularly adamant about receiving the mixture of Mercurochrome and hydrogen peroxide. This was a favorite for just about everything, probably because of the bright red color.

If an abscess was runny, sulfur powder was sprinkled on. The powder was expensive and not always available, in which case expired bottles of penicillin powder were torn open and used as a substitute.

The emphasis was always on making do—if it can't hurt, give it a try. It was the spirit that counted. The faith of these nuns could bend physical laws and make miracles. Especially the miracle of love that Mother Teresa taught them: "Be kind and merciful. Let no one ever come to you without leaving better and happier. Be the living expression of God's kindness; kindness in your face, kindness in your eyes, kindness in your smile, kindness in your warm greeting. In the slums we are the light of God's kindness to the poor. To children, to the poor, to all who suffer and are lonely, give always a happy smile. Give them not only your care, but also your heart."

We didn't see many old people in Port-au-Prince. We were told by the Sisters that the mortality rate from birth to five years was 50 percent. The average life span was twenty-five to thirty years. But one of the regulars appeared to be a fairly old man, very thin, with a twisted and misshapen left arm.

The arm was full of abscesses, with a large open sore in the elbow area. The man was suffering from an advanced stage of syphilis. He begged the nuns to help him get the arm cut off. After a time they agreed to assist with the amputation. Arrangements were made at the community hospital. It was quite a feat to set it up, including finding a willing doctor, but the nuns had many connections along with their strong determination, will and prayer. Beds were not assigned at the hospital so the nuns had to scout around and find one—making a quick claim on the spot. Further, no food or medication was given out; every patient had to have his or her own supply.

After all was made ready, the old man had his arm amputated. We didn't see him for a few days. When he showed up again he looked cheerful and grinned proudly, displaying a stump that extended four or five inches from his shoulder. He came regularly as usual, for dressing changes. The stump never healed. The abscess set in deeper and he became weaker. He was ill and dying and received little reprieve. His countenance was resigned and he never complained. His gentle smile remained to the very end.

The hospital procedure was too complex for the average illiterate native to negotiate. Many who went for treatment were too weak to leave, had no one there to assist them, and were removed to a shack behind the hospital called the depot. There, they were left to their own resources or lack thereof.

The depot consisted of a dirt floor, walls to lean against, and a roof to keep the rain out. When the Sisters of Charity first arrived in Haiti they arranged for the hospital to deliver these outcasts to their home for the ill and dying, but they themselves had to go to the depot each day to see who was there and what their needs were. Then they would go to the hospital administration and request a delivery. One of the first people they encountered in the beginning was a young man who was paralyzed from the neck down. They were too late to retrieve him. Rats had eaten him while he was still alive.

I went to the depot once with Sister Jacqueline. There were two rooms opening in back to an old outhouse. Two men were lying on mats in the first room. Sister stopped and spoke with them. In the back room was an old woman on a cot. Sister explained to me that she was paralyzed and her family no longer wanted her in their home. They did, however, pay someone to bring her food and change her each day.

The Sisters did what they could. They tried to offer, in their home for the ill and dying destitute, a place where people could face death with dignity and the comfort of love. The home was overflowing. Cots spilled outdoors and lined the walkways. The Sisters had to discriminate. Not all of the ill and dying poor could be accommodated. As Mother Teresa expressed it:

> We ourselves feel that what we are doing is just a drop in the ocean. But if that drop was not in the ocean, I think the ocean would be less because of that missing drop. I do not agree with the big way of doing things. To us what matters is an individual. To get to love the person we must come in close contact with him. If we wait till we get the numbers, then we will be lost in the numbers. And we will never be able to show that love and respect for the person. I believe in person to person; every person is

Christ for me, and since there is only one Jesus, that person is the one person in the world at that moment.

In the scabies section where I spent much of my time, we witnessed an unending cycle. There were no facilities for proper hygiene, and because we couldn't speak the language fluently we made little progress in our attempts to educate people in self-care. Two of us would set up in the morning with two plastic basins of water. On some days there was enough water to change the basins once during the course of the morning's work, but more often the water we started with was the same water we ended with. Countless babies and mothers, children, and a few fathers shared each basin. Staff members generally had one towel each and a metal box with our supplies: a special medicated shampoo, Isodine for cleaning, cotton swabs, Mercurochrome, Kwell (a commercial ointment containing DDT that was used to eliminate scabies), and a mild skin lotion.

Scabies are little animals similar to ticks or chiggers that burrow under the skin. They are spread by touching affected skin or through contact with infested clothes and bedding. Scratching causes infection and produces little sores with pus. We treated people whose bodies were covered with these sores. The scabies concentrate particularly between the toes and fingers, under the breasts of females, around the cracks of the buttocks, and on the private parts of both males and females. The itching is agonizing.

Most often we would treat mothers and infants, knowing we were not getting to the whole family or addressing the problem of contaminated clothing and bedding. After treatment we used our limited Creole to tell them not to wash that day but to wash well the next day with soap and water. We knew most of them had no soap and the water they had access to was most likely gutter water.

The first person I worked on was a young woman who lived on the streets. Her entire body was covered with small abscessed sores. She was feverish and weak. The blue dress she was wearing looked as though it had never been washed, except perhaps by the rain. She had no shoes and no underclothes. Her body smelled not only of sweat but of decaying tissue, an odor we grew accustomed to at the clinic. She was small, quiet, sweet-faced, and complied humbly when I asked her to remove her dress. Her buttocks were a continuous scab. There was not an unmarked spot on her body. With gloved hands I washed her and shampooed her hair, applied Mercurochrome to her sores and Kwell everywhere except on her hair and the delicate tissues of her face.

The girl showed up regularly, and I cleaned her sores and helped as much as I could. One day she showed up so ill and feverish that she was too weak to stand. An American priest had arrived that day and was working with me. When I told him her history, he asked that I keep her there while he went off to his room to retrieve one of the dresses he had brought with him, gifts collected by his parishioners for the poor. I managed to remove the blue dress, which by now was as stiff as cardboard, and helped her into the new one the priest offered.

I tossed the stiff garment into a corner, telling the girl I would wash it. I was busy with a long line of people waiting for treatment, and when I turned my attention back to where the girl had been resting, she was gone. So was the old blue dress.

At the end of the day the priest came and apologetically told me he was leaving in the morning. The conditions were too unbearable for him. I remembered a time several years earlier when I had accepted a job at a rest home and worked the night shift. At one o'clock we had to make rounds, going into rooms and switching on bright overhead lights, waking people up and subjecting them to an invasion of privacy while we checked their bedding and bodies to see if they needed changing. In the morning I combed through the tangled silver hair of one of my charges before wheeling her to the breakfast room. Tears of gratitude spilled down her cheeks for that simple attention. When I got home I burst into tears and couldn't stop crying. By afternoon I called and quit. I understood very well how the priest was feeling.

One day as I was walking through an outdoor market, I looked up and saw the young girl walking toward me wearing her blue dress. We exchanged greetings and I asked her how she was. She answered with a shy smile and nod. Her skin was scarred but looked much better.

A few weeks later I was working in the scabies room and looked up to see a nun helping a young girl in a blue dress into the room. She had been found lying in the street, too weak to get up. Her skin was as infected as it had been the first time I saw her. I felt the futility of this vicious cycle and remembered what Peace Pilgrim had said when we told her we were coming to Haiti to work.

"I myself work on the causes of suffering, but I bless those who work on symptoms." Then shaking her head she had continued, "You'll find conditions that are symptoms of greed and exploitation. Hunger and poverty are actually symptoms of symptoms." I hadn't stopped to consider what she meant, but now I was seeing firsthand. We would clean this young woman's sores again, offer temporary comfort and relief, and send her back to the conditions that caused her suffering.

Once again I managed to get her into a clean dress and even gave her an extra blouse to take with her. It would undoubtedly be sold, as the first dress we had put her in had been. But this time I confiscated the stiff blue dress, now in tatters, and took it to another room where I buried it unceremoniously under the garbage in a wastebasket. It was easy to feel that the situation was hopeless; but I also knew that someone had to feed and clothe these people until enough of us who had the means and education could diligently address the cause of this terrible suffering.

The causes of this gross imbalance were all around me. Large, mostly American companies had control over big parcels of land. These companies had resources that could have been used to foster self-reliance in the local population, training people to grow the nutritious food they so desperately needed. Instead, the companies were using up precious water supplies to grow tobacco and sugar cane, paying wages that kept the people impoverished.

Dotted throughout Port-au-Prince were islands of lush green

landscaping behind walls that housed tourist hotels. In contrast, a cardboard shack where people took turns sleeping in shifts stood on bare earth baked hard by the sun. The shack stood near a home surrounded by a high iron fence. It was the only real house in that area. As with the hotels, I could look through the bars at lush green plants and trees laden with tropical fruits. Only once did I see a person, no doubt a maid, with eyes cast down and a basket of fruit under her arm, scurry into the door and out of sight.

Despite the poverty and disease, the gaiety of the people and the grace with which they moved stood out. A rhythmic pulse seemed to beat at the heart of the culture, even reverberating in the beat of voodoo drums when the sun went down.

We might have felt some shyness or guilt about our perceived status or white skin, but any such feelings were laid to rest after our first ride on local transportation. As we stood conspicuously among a group of black people clamoring to get aboard a tap-tap (a van that opened from the back and had benches running along the sides) people good-naturedly stepped back as eager hands reached out to pull the three of us inside.

We were pushed into seats, and all eyes fixed on us. A. Z., wearing shorts, looked around and then down at his bare legs. A couple of women started to giggle. He looked at them and in a serious voice asked if they were looking at his legs. He picked one up and waved it around as he continued speaking English, still looking serious. Without understanding a word he was saying, the entire bus was soon laughing and having a gay time. I don't think one person got off until we did. Two women followed us a short distance and then ran up and pulled my hair from behind. Startled at first, I looked around and they burst into giggles, covering their mouths. I laughed too, guessing that my smooth straight hair was intriguing to them.

Another time the two Andys and I were at the big market square where we shopped regularly, when some of the women sellers started pointing at me and asking questions. We didn't understand, but A. Z. indicated through gestures that the three of us were together. They must have been asking which of the two of them was my husband, because they seemed to get the idea that I was married to both of them. A great ruckus broke out, and women from all over the market began following and cheering me. Faces lit up whenever we came into the market after that. I can only imagine what stories we generated.

Back at the clinic Andy had taken charge of the TB patients and directed the giving of injections on Saturdays. The banana lady, a merchant we always bought from at the market, was a Saturday regular. It was obvious that her familiarity with us gave her some status, and one morning she boldly pushed her way to the front of the line. Andy saw what she had done and, picking up a foot-long demonstration model of a syringe, pointed it at her, indicating that he planned to use this one on her if she didn't go back to the end of the line. She got his point and in mock fear threw her arms up and ran to the end of the line screaming, while the crowd cheered and laughed.

During our stay groups of Americans would come for three-week periods, usually sponsored by a church. Very often the groups would include a nurse, a priest, a dentist or doctor, and five or six others with varying backgrounds. We enjoyed many new acquaintances and friends from among the visiting workers; a bonding of kinship and fellowship developed naturally among us. In these dramatic circumstances, people often left with a positive feeling of having participated in something very special.

We established a close working relationship with a dentist named John and his wife, Sue, who expressed this sentiment well in a letter she wrote to us later:

> John went back to his office and I went back to my work with the mentally retarded. The month in Haiti has never left our consciousness, however, and you must know that our mission trips influence whatever we do. The seven years in mission work did not compare with this last year. In other years we saw poverty

but it was rural—in the mountains or the jungles. Poverty in Port-au-Prince was different. The crowded conditions, the filth, and the disease were so tremendous this year. We were lucky to have such good companions during our stay. That too, was new to us, because we had always worked alone. Living together in a communal setting with seven strangers could be dreadful but, in this instance, it was beautiful. There was never a cross word or an argument.

We all benefited from the privilege of working together, although the Andys and I didn't live in the complex with the others where the limited space was better used for short-term volunteers. Two days after arriving we had found a monthly rental at L'Habitation Hatt, a complex of apartments. Our unit was like a townhouse, with a small living room and kitchen downstairs, and a bedroom and bathroom upstairs. The only furnishings were A. Z.'s sleeping mat tucked under the staircase downstairs and the two mats in the bedroom upstairs. The staircase itself substituted for chairs.

Despite the fact that we had arrived in January, the weather remained hot and humid. My legs would feel like lead when we trudged home at the end of the day, sweat rolling down our faces and soaking our clothes. The sisters assured us that this was the most pleasant time of year. By summer they described how several times a day they stopped to slip out of their saris and wring them out before putting them back on.

We called the last incline on the road home "the grinder." From the top of the hill we could see the wet, shimmering blue of water. Within minutes we would luxuriate in the refreshingly cool and heavily chlorinated swimming pool. It became a place of refuge for us and our coworkers at the end of the day. It was where we gathered to "disinfect," as we jokingly called it, after a day's work among the sick and dying.

POVERTY'S CHILDREN

As with the dispensary, on the days we worked at the children's home we would arrive just before eight. We entered through a back gate, went through a courtyard where native women in blue uniforms were already busy washing clothes in large tubs of water, and climbed the stairs. Here, we would pause while our eyes adjusted to the dimness of the inner rooms.

Ahead of us was an L-shaped corridor with painted walls and cement floors. The first room on the left was the kitchen and pantry. Straight ahead was a room where the older children slept. As the corridor turned to the right, there was a large room that opened into an alcove facing the street. This room contained a picnic table where the children often played.

Two more rooms opened off the corridor and were filled with cribs and beds. We called the first one the sick room. It was where the most seriously ill were placed. The second we called the baby room as it housed the smallest children. Many of them looked like infants, but the children were actually up to four years old. A smile might reveal a full set of teeth.

The first time I walked into this room, my eyes were still adjusting to the dimness as I glanced at an emaciated child propped up in a sitting position against a wall. I saw some movement in front of him and his hand reached out to pick something up. He put it to his mouth and just as I heard the loud crunch my eyes focused more clearly: it was a two-inch long cockroach.

We had to walk very carefully when proceeding down the hallway. In the dimness it would be easy to step on one of the tiny bodies that lay curled up on the bare floor, some asleep and others with eyes open in a staring gaze. We also wanted to avoid stepping in the little piles and wet spots left by not yet potty-trained children who either had not been diapered or had managed to slip out of a hastily tied diaper. The floors were washed thoroughly once each day, usually after breakfast, but were soon littered again. After that the workers, not trained in cleanliness or hygiene, cleaned them as time or inclination allowed.

We would go to the baby room first to check if breakfast was underway yet. A small table in the corner held a large bowl filled with cereal and small bowls stacked around it, along with plastic spoons. If there was time we would make a quick survey of the room, changing the most obviously dirty diapers.

Then feeding would begin in an assembly line fashion. Babies who could sit up were lined against a wall. Bowls of cereal with spoons were placed in front of them and a worker would squat down and scoot through the line depositing a spoonful of food in each mouth. There was no time for fussiness. Babies swallowed fast and opened their mouths for the next pass. The weaker or smaller ones who remained in cribs lay on their backs and were fed individually. What didn't go in, as spoonfuls came at them in rapid succession, dripped down the front of them.

When the babies had been fed we would go to the sick room to help with the feeding there. I flinched every time I saw a worker place a spoonful of food into one sick child's mouth and then proceed to another child, placing the same spoon in his or her mouth. Malnutrition was not the only ailment being treated. The children suffered from typhoid, TB, dysentery, and a large variety of fevers and germs. The head nun often chided the workers and tried to correct their bad habits. The workers would listen and nod their heads in acknowledgment, and then smilingly continue as before.

When the older children finished their meal on the back covered porch, they would wander in with smiles and giggles and sometimes tears. They were mostly a jolly, motley crew of ragamuffins. They would throw their arms around our legs, plead to be picked up, pull on us, and converge to swarm us if we ever sat down.

With the first feeding over, workers would shuttle the older children out to the courtyard where they lined up and waited for morning showers. Inside, we would move the little table from the baby room to the corridor in front of a shelf that was filled with clothes and powder and ointments. One worker would kneel next to a small tub of heated water while we went around collecting babies. Starting in the baby room we would pick up a dirty child, remove its diaper and top, and deposit it in the waiting worker's arms. She would pour water over the child, then suds it from head to toe before pouring water over it again. The squalling child would then be handed to one of us to soothe and powder and dress.

It was my favorite time. For at least this moment each day all the babies smelled good and were clean. Boys got a T-shirt, girls a dress, and everyone got a diaper. There were never enough clothes of the proper fit, so most of the children wore garments that hung from their tiny frames.

Sister Georgia, a figure of stability and loving warmth, was in charge of the children's home. The workers tended to the children's needs, but I didn't see many displays of affection. Sister Georgia, in contrast, beamed love. She had the utmost patience with the children, even the special ones who could be very tiresome and difficult.

One such retarded boy was about twelve years old, tall and lanky. Sister told us he had been born normal; his retardation was the result of a beating by his father. When he had first arrived he was unable to even walk. Sister had manipulated his arms and legs until he was able to get up and move about by himself. When we met him he wore a diaper and followed the other children around. His coordination was poor, his intellect severely limited, and he was often a target for the other children's frustrations. Before we left, his family came and took him home.

Though I tried to be impartial, I couldn't help developing favorites among the children. My heart will always flutter at the memory of Maxi. Maxi came in one day, a beautiful boy about six years of age, with an angelic face. His body was thin though not as emaciated as some. His expression was forlorn. The workers had little patience or empathy for the new arrivals. They rather rigorously indoctrinated them into the routine from the beginning. My heart went out to the little boy and, feeling my concern, he stuck very close to me that day.

When I was busy feeding the babies or dressing them, he would stand beside me and hold onto my leg. When I wasn't busy I would hold him and give him hugs.

I didn't realize at first that the workers took exception to my special treatment of him. I began to notice that when my back was turned they would poke at Maxi and whisper. Whenever possible they would force him away to another room. They were harsher on him than they would have been if he had not clung to me and if I had not encouraged it. As the days went by I learned to be more subtle in demonstrating my affections.

I continued to adore Maxi and I knew he understood. For a while he tried to manipulate me by pouting whenever I showed up. When that failed to get my attention or approval, he turned flirtatious and irresistible. With the language barrier we communicated through facial expression and touch. He adjusted well to his life at the home and became a natural leader among the children.

The home was a temporary placement center for sick and malnourished children, not an orphanage, and on Sundays special clothes were brought out for greeting visiting parents. I will always remember Maxi's face as it beamed one Sunday morning when we uncovered a bright red top with matching shorts to dress him in.

We nicknamed another special child "Sleeper." The first time we saw him he was sitting on the floor with his face tilted upward, eyes closed in sleep; he was rocking back and forth. When he was awake he would sit in the same position, observing the world with his head tilted back and a grin on his face. After a while, as he began to recognize us, his arm would fly up in a one-arm salute, the grin on his face extending from ear to ear. In time his one-arm greeting evolved into a two-arm salute and his smile filled my heart.

On another day a beautiful little girl named Michelle arrived. Her hair had the reddish blond color that is one of the signs of malnutrition in black children. Her little body was emaciated, and she was so ill and weak at first that she had to be fed through a tube down her throat. At three and a half years old, she was the size of an infant.

She would lie quietly in her crib each day, her face expressionless.

After she had been in the home long enough to gain some strength, I picked her up and carried her with me while I went around visiting other children. We even sat on the floor of the bathroom and watched Andy work on a broken pipe. The next day when we came in, I caught her eye as I surveyed the room, and her face lit up in a beautiful smile. It was the first of many. In time she was sitting up and even feeding herself.

The cycle of poverty and disease is hard to break and on some days it seemed futile. Yet even at the children's home, sounds of bright laughter rang out in sharp contrast to the dark dimness of the inner rooms. Children romped in brightly colored tattered clothing down the halls, while others filled rows of beds, ravaged with fevers or weak from dysentery or TB. Some lived and some died. It was with a mixture of sadness and relief, sometimes, that we would witness little bodies that had known only struggle give up their pain and succumb to death. The tiniest was buried in a shoe box.

It was easy to slip into the pervading belief that we were somehow privileged and invulnerable to the poverty and disease all around us. We drank bottled water and bought and prepared our food carefully. I remember a particular American volunteer who arrived with all her own food, prepared to eat nothing fresh for the three-week period she planned on staying. We all laughed when I offered her a banana and she shook her head adamantly, reminding me she intended to be extra careful. At the end of the first week she came down with a fever that landed her in bed for several days. After that I noticed her eating bananas.

The Andys and I had been in Haiti for more than two months when A. Z. became ill. He took to his cot under the stairway with typhoid fever. It was the first crack in my sense of personal invulnerability. A. Z. had incredible physical and psychological endurance, but as I watched him slip in and out of delirium I saw how close death could come to any of us. I was gratefully relieved when he recovered.

FACE TO FACE WITH MORTALITY

A short time later we had a sort of dinner party for a group of our American friends. It was a night of disinfecting in the pool and enjoying what we dubbed "Haitian stew"—a medley of eggplant and whatever vegetables we could get at the market.

I had been noticing a pain in my head for some time, and this night it reached a crescendo. I left the party to crawl under my mosquito netting upstairs. One of our friends, an American doctor, followed me up. She confirmed what I suspected: I had come down with viral meningitis, a fever of the brain. The discomfort increased until it became impossible to move even my eyeballs without excruciating pain. Days passed as I lay feverish on my mat. I elected not to go to a Haitian hospital, assuring the Andys that I would be all right left alone while they worked. Then one afternoon I was overcome by a wave of loneliness and melancholy. I felt far from home and my heart ached to see my daughter. Cindy, who was with my brother and sister-in-law in Arizona, seemed worlds away.

I was suddenly startled by a chorus of voices behind me, each voice intoning my name in a fantastic harmony. Before I could even react, a single voice called my name commandingly. I was instantly drawn out of my body through the top of my head and upward to a cloudlike resting place, where I could just barely hear the chorus echoing my name fade out. The pain was completely gone. I was aware of brilliant light, although there was no glare, and an indescribable, all-encompassing peace. It was as if the very substance of the space was embracing me in unconditional love and gentleness.

After a moment I noticed an opening below me; looking down, I recognized the United States. Then—as if I was being spoken to in a voice but without words, as if a thought of my own had come to me from the outside—I was clearly told that that was where my work was. I was entranced with the brilliant peacefulness surrounding me. I silently asked or thought, "Can't I just stay here?" I was instantly thrust back into my body with a jarring resurgence of pain. As I opened my eyes I saw a bird hovering in the window the way hummingbirds do, although it was much larger, and then it flew away. This seemed somehow significant. Perhaps the sense of being observed further confirmed what I had experienced.

That afternoon when the Andys came home, I told them what had happened. I asked them to feel the palms of my hands, which felt like burning circles of heat, as did the center of my forehead just above my eyes. One of them touched my palm and said, "It's hot enough to fry an egg on!" I drifted in and out of consciousness as my fever peaked. My husband sat up with me all night, holding my head in his lap and comforting me.

By morning my temperature had dropped to slightly below normal and, except for weakness, I felt well. I was able to get up and shower for the first time since the illness began. I was barely out of the shower when I heard a knock on the door downstairs. It was a group of Mother Teresa's nuns, demanding to take me to the hospital. I went down the stairs and stood in the middle of the room while a dozen little women in white saris circled around me. "Cherril, ve take you to de hospital," Sister Carmeline, the head nun, stated emphatically. But I told them the fever was gone. They looked at me in disbelief, as did my friend the American doctor, when I went back to work the following day. "I must have made a mistake in my diagnosis," she stated. "Otherwise, you couldn't possibly be well."

But well I was, and very aware that I had come back from death's door. With all the death and illness I had witnessed among the Haitians, my understanding of what they felt had now shifted from observation to participation. I had also learned much about myself. Coming from a society where many people are ill-prepared to accept their own mortality, I felt that I had come to terms with my own. I had never really feared death, and now I could actually look forward to it as a beautiful experience when the time came.

The vision from my near-death experience had a strong impact. I would be forever grateful for all I had seen and experienced in Haiti, but I knew it was time to return home to the United States.

14

The Greatest Gift

True teaching liberates the student from his teacher.
He will find the teacher within himself.

ERNEST HOLMES

It was nearly summer and beautiful in the hills above Phoenix, where Andy and I had settled into a comfortable routine and Cindy was finishing her last year of high school. I made weekly pilgrimages to the majestic red rocks and forests surrounding Prescott Valley, walked around Lynx Lake, and discovered magical places off the beaten path. Peace had written to me about two retreats she was planning to lead in Pennsylvania later in the year and asked if I could join her to help out. I sent my enthusiastic agreement by return mail.

I was excited to tell Peace about our adventures in Haiti, and there were many questions I had for her. I waited in happy anticipation for an answer to my letter, but none came. Instead, a month later, I received a letter that started, "Have you received the sad news of Peace Pilgrim? She was killed in an auto accident a month ago."

DEALING WITH GRIEF

The idea was simply inconceivable. I wanted to believe it was a mistake. How could it be true? I was overcome with grief. Spending so much time with Peace over the past few years had helped me forge a sense of direction and rightness about life. Now a part of me felt lost.

At work the next day I couldn't stop the tears from spilling down my cheeks. I was sent home with kind words to take as much time as I needed. It felt as though everything I thought I knew had broken into pieces, and I needed to figure out how to put it all back together.

My thoughts kept going back to the islands I had visited with Peace. Two days later I was on a plane heading for Maui. At the airport I rented a car, and a few miles away I found a little cottage for lease across the street from the ocean. I rented it. After unloading my bag, I drove back to the airport to turn the car in and walk "home."

The cottage I had chosen was nestled in a private little cove, with an aromatic plumeria tree on one side of the porch and a papaya tree on the other. Every morning I would go out and pick a fresh plumeria blossom for my hair from one tree and a papaya for breakfast from the other.

One day melted into another as I roamed in solitude on white sandy beaches that stretched for miles in either direction. Every morning I would go out needing only a bathing suit and shorts in the mild balmy weather, and carrying fresh fruit and water. In the late afternoon I would carry home groceries and supplies from a small store in a nearby town.

LESSONS START COMING

I was sitting at a picnic table on a beach enjoying the shade under a tree one afternoon when I noticed an injured bird. Its wing was twisted and it sat awkwardly on the ground. It seemed heartless to just leave it there, but I resisted taking on the responsibility of caring for it. *I can't take it with me, I don't have anything to carry it in*, I said to myself.

Then I noticed a cardboard box nearby. *Well, cardboard is so smooth and slippery, and there's nothing to cover the bottom with*. As soon as I finished the thought, I saw a patch of grass in the sand that would make good bedding. Still resisting, I thought, *I have no idea what the bird eats*.

It would starve if I took it home. On cue, the bird struggled to reach one of the many pods full of seeds that had fallen from the tree and were scattered in profusion on the ground.

Recognizing that I was out of excuses I started to accept the idea of taking the little bird home with me. As I surrendered my resistance, the bird looked at me, stood on its feet, and gracefully straightening its crumpled wing, flew away.

As I watched in surprise, I was reminded of a story Peace had told. It had taken place during a period of prayer and fasting that she had undertaken for forty days. While in a state between wakefulness and sleep, she had a vision of a dismal cross above her and understood that someone had to take up the burden. When she reached up to accept it, she was lifted above the cross where all was beauty and light. All that had been needed was her willingness to accept the burden, and she was raised above it. I knew I'd gotten a big lesson from the bird.

I walked along the beach for miles, enjoying the warmth of the sand under my feet and mulling over the principles and ideals Peace had talked about and demonstrated. I knew how powerful her teachings were; I also knew how challenging it was to really live my beliefs. Part of me was still a doubting Thomas, thinking that these higher spiritual laws worked only for saints or sages. While I struggled to understand intellectually, the universe moved in its own way, creating the experiences I needed to test my convictions and forcing me to confront my fears.

One test was fairly simple. As I walked on a quiet stretch of beach, a barking dog came out of the trees in the distance, charging at me. All I could do was stand my ground, using the commanding attitude Peace had demonstrated in Alaska (admittedly with less authority than she had shown) but the dog stopped in its tracks and walked away. This small feat perhaps gave me the courage to confront my next and biggest test.

As I walked along a remote dirt road early one morning, I noticed three large native men moving toward me. They were walking with the kind of swagger a friend laughingly called "the macho walk."

They were speaking loudly, and their voices carried in the breeze. With a sick feeling I realized they were talking about molesting me.

I knew I couldn't run away, and even if I tried they would easily overtake me. Fear rose up in my chest. At the same time I heard the words Peace had spoken when talking about the little girl she had defended: "You attract to you the very thing that you fear, and I knew the girl was in great danger."

Immediately I began to imagine lifting the fear up out of my body. Then I imagined lifting myself and the three men into God's hands. As I let go, knowing I couldn't control the situation or the outcome, a calmness took over. When the men were close enough, I made eye contact with each of them and, in the cheeriest voice I could muster, I said, "Good morning!"

The men who had seemed so scary suddenly looked like three schoolboys. Their eyes dropped to the ground, and they stumbled over their feet, mumbling "Good morning," in response.

Their reaction took me totally by surprise. I walked by without looking back. I hadn't expected to walk away unharmed. "No one walks more safely than one who walks humbly and lovingly," Peace's voice echoed, "for they reach the good in the other person and the person is disarmed."

MAKING SENSE OF DEATH

Following this powerful demonstration of protection, my mind went to the seeming tragedy of Peace's death. How could Peace, who felt such protection around her, have been killed by a car in a head-on collision?

Then I remembered how Peace's face lit up when she recounted her own near-death experience. She had been walking in the high mountains of Arizona when a surprising snowstorm came out of season:

> I was walking in a very isolated area, and I knew there was no human habitation for many miles. That afternoon there came one

of those quick snowstorms. If it had been rain you would have called it a cloudburst, the snow just piled up so quickly. I noticed that the cars had stopped running on the road because they were getting stuck in the snow. And right after that, darkness descended. Total darkness. I couldn't even see my hand before my eyes. The snow was blowing in my face and it was bitter cold. It was the kind of cold that penetrates into the marrow of your bones.

If ever I were to lose faith and feel fear, certainly this should have been the time. But instead this whole experience of the cold and the snow and the darkness seemed to be unreal, to be an illusion. And the only thing that seemed real to me in that situation was the awareness of the presence of God. At that moment I knew that I was not this transient body. I knew that I was the indestructible reality that activates this body. When you identify not with the destructible clay garment but with the indestructible reality, how free you feel. I knew everything was going to be all right whether I remained to serve in this Earth life or whether I went on to serve in a freer life beyond.

I felt guided to keep on walking. I couldn't see if I was walking along that highway or out into some field. I couldn't see anything. My feet in my low canvas shoes were like lumps of ice. They just felt so heavy as I plodded along. Then my whole body began to become numb with the cold. When there was more numbness than pain, there came what some would refer to as a hallucination and what some would refer to as a vision. It was as though I became aware not only of the embodied side of life, where everything was black darkness and bitter cold and swirling snow, but also—and it seemed so close I could step right over into it, indeed it is right here in another dimension—the unembodied side of life where everything was warm and light.

There was great beauty. It began with familiar color, and yet it transcended familiar color. Maybe that's what the artists see. I became aware of what began as familiar music but transcended familiar music. Perhaps that's what the musicians hear. Then I saw beings, way off at a great distance, a lot of them, but only one moved toward me. She moved quickly, and when she came within ten or twelve feet of me I recognized my aunt, although she looked much younger than she had looked when she had stepped over. And since I believe that at the time of the beginning of the change called death those nearest and dearest come to welcome us—I've been with those who stepped over and I remember well how they talked to their loved ones on both sides as though they were all right there in the room together—I thought my time had come to step over. I greeted her and I either said or thought to her, "You've come for me?" But she shook her head and motioned for me to go back.

And just at that point I ran into the railing of a bridge and the vision faded. Then because I felt guided to do so, I groped my way down that snowy embankment and under that bridge I found a large cardboard packing box. And it was full of wrapping paper. And very slowly and clumsily in my numb condition, I managed to get myself inside of that packing box. And somehow with my numb fingers I managed to pull that wrapping paper around me. And there, under the bridge during the snowstorm, I slept. Even there shelter had been provided.

But provided also had been this experience. Had you looked at me in the midst of it you might have said, "What a difficult experience that poor woman is going through." But looking back on it I can only say what a wonderful experience, in which I faced death feeling not fear but the constant awareness of the presence of God, which you take right over with you. And of course I believe that I have had the great privilege of experiencing the beginning of the change called death. What a beautiful experience. And now I can rejoice with my loved ones as they make the glorious transition to a freer living.

My grief started to lift as I recalled her story. I could imagine her surrounded by angels at the time of her transition, and reaching out as her loved ones approached, asking again, "Have you come for me?" Death is, after all, an experience we all face at the end of life's journey. I remembered the unconditional love and peace I had felt during my own near-death experience. I still felt sadness at the loss of Peace's physical presence, but it was softer now; I was able to embrace it in a way that was comforting.

And then a great realization came. In dying, Peace had left the greatest gift of all. It was the reminder to look within. All the questions I had been waiting to ask her I was now asking inside. And, as I listened in the stillness, the answers were coming. Intellectually I had understood when Peace talked about the teacher within: "Don't look to me. Look to your own inner teacher." But I had continued to put questions aside to ask her. Now that she was gone I was reconnecting to that inner source. I was ready to return home.

15

More Good-byes

Death confounds us with its timing and its apparent disregard of human plans and hopes; the ending of a relationship may similarly throw us into endless wonder about its meaning.

THOMAS MOORE

A memorial service was held for Peace, and many of her friends from all over the country were invited. For two weeks people came and went, sharing memories, personal letters, tapes of her talks, and photographs. Many people expressed a desire to see her work and words carried on, and several individuals toyed with the idea of writing a book about her life.

When the crowds dwindled five of us were left. As we discussed the impact that Peace's life had had on so many people, we came to the conclusion that no one could tell her story better than she did herself. Hundreds of newspaper articles chronicling Peace's pilgrimage had been gathered and stored in the Peace Archives at Swarthmore College, and even more stories and talks had surfaced at the memorial. There was more than enough material to compile into a book in her own words. Richard Polese, Ann and John Rush, A. Z., and I decided to take the project on ourselves.

Peace Pilgrim's life, like that of saints of old, had been more like the mythical tale of a traveling angel. "Enjoy the seasons of life," she had advised, "they are short." Seasons come and go, and so it is with life. There are individuals whose passing becomes obscured in time. Others leave behind an intangible essence, an inspiration that enters the hearts of even those who have never met them. And so it was with Peace, whose key to a vibrant life was the joy of giving her own life in service.

In a few short weeks our concentrated efforts produced the first draft of a book called *Peace Pilgrim: Her Life and Work in Her Own Words*. It was published less than one year after her death and, with more than five hundred thousand copies currently in print, continues to touch and inspire people.

EMBARKING ON A CROSS-COUNTRY TREK

After the book was completed I wasn't ready to close that chapter of my life. I made plans to walk across the country from San Francisco to Washington, D.C., so that I could experience more of what Peace's life had been like. Both Andy and A. Z. embraced the idea, and as word got around we were contacted by several others who wanted to join us.

There were a myriad of details to work out before the departure date from San Francisco on Easter Sunday. Richard helped me put together news releases. I plotted a route and timetable across the country, locating post offices where we could pick up mail addressed to general delivery. A. Z. retrieved an old pop-up travel trailer he had stored away and attached it to his station wagon; this became our support vehicle. Andy and my father designed and built an ingenious fiberglass pop-up toilet that folded down behind the trailer for less wind resistance. A big sign extending the length of the car was erected on the roof. It read, "PRAYER FOR PEACE PILGRIMAGE."

We weren't traveling as simply as Peace, who'd walked with only the clothes she was wearing, but, as she said, people's needs are different. It was basic enough for our purposes. The support vehicle enabled us to walk unencumbered and have our gear waiting at the end of the day. Because this walk was commemorating Peace, I designed navy blue vests for the participants with white lettering that read, "ANOTHER PILGRIM FOR PEACE" on the front and "WALKING COAST TO COAST FOR PEACE" on the back.

A few days before departure, the group started gathering at a beach in Half Moon Bay, the designated meeting place near San Francisco. Two men and the only other woman slated to come didn't show up, leaving me with a group of five men. Others were planning to join us at various points along the way.

The day before departure we moved camp to an RV park in San Francisco, and Andy and I spent our last day walking around downtown. We stood out in the lettered vests; it was easy to see why Peace had chosen this approach to meeting people. The reactions we encountered were generally positive and curious. People asked what we were doing and wished us well. A man who was panhandling on a corner spotted us and started heading our way. I involuntarily drew back, mentally preparing myself to politely turn him down when he approached. But instead of asking for money, he enthusiastically offered us five dollars.

On Easter morning we woke up to pouring rain after a restless night filled with the sounds of a frantic windstorm. The sun came out as we drove to our departure point at the New Windmill in Golden Gate Park. Several friends and relatives carpooled to the site and walked with us to the conservatory, where we had arranged to have an Easter Service. After a picnic lunch we said good-bye and began the three-thousand-mile journey.

I looked back at my daughter, Cindy, looking young and vulnerable in the distance. Recently married, she had just discovered she was pregnant with her first child, and now this walk would keep me away until she was well into her third trimester. I felt the tightness in my chest that would be a continuing reminder of the conflict I felt at being pulled in two directions.

In both purpose and structure, the walk was to be an opportunity to demonstrate peace by putting the principles of peace into practice in as many ways as we could. We all agreed, for example, to find peaceful ways to resolve any conflicts that might come up among us in the intensity of living so closely together. We even designated one side of the road for silence so anyone could have some space and quiet time alone when he or she wanted it. Another objective was to meet with other individuals and groups and speak with them on the topic of peace. Toward that end we carried a brochure telling about our walk and gave out a little booklet called *Steps Toward Inner Peace*, transcribed from a talk given by Peace Pilgrim. As on the retreats with Peace, the fare was vegetarian, and all participants agreed not to use alcohol, drugs, or nicotine.

A. Z. came up with an idea to demonstrate peace with the environment by picking up aluminum cans, which we did all the way from San Francisco to Washington, D.C. We cashed the cans in at recycling centers along the way and made enough money to pay for all the gas and maintenance for our support vehicle. There was even enough left over for us to stay at an official campground once a week where we could get a hot shower whether, as we would joke, we needed it or not.

I had learned a lot of practical things from Peace about living outdoors, and I became quite adept at finding ways to stay clean. When facilities weren't available, I filled a large tin can with water and in the privacy of the little pop-up toilet took a sponge bath and washed out my underclothes. Also, because I was often the only woman, when we were offered hospitality along the way (we were frequently invited to dinner or to talk to a group or given a place to park at night), I was almost always offered a shower and shampoo—even when "the boys" were not. I felt a little guilty, but not so much that I didn't accept and enjoy it.

Each of us contributed twenty dollars a week to the community pot for food and supplies and, in Peace Pilgrim style, didn't accept donations. When money was offered we explained that our walk was for peace and it was our intention to inspire others to find ways to work for peace in their own lives and communities. We asked people to join us in our prayer for peace and to look to prayer as a means of inspiration leading to meaningful action. What seemed like a simple gesture touched people more deeply than we could have imagined, as all along the way our appeal brought people to tears. When we wouldn't take money, we were often given food or supplies or shown some other hospitality, and we gratefully accepted what was offered.

Eleven days after leaving San Francisco, we reached Lake Tahoe and our first two day break. We had slept in parking lots, parks, one official campground, an old train yard, and various other sites along the road. It was all I could do to make it up the last long hill into Tahoe. The first day out, my feet had gotten wet in puddles from the rain, and a blister now covered the bottom of one heel. Favoring that foot had thrown my back out, so I couldn't bend over. My hands and face were covered with a rash from sun poisoning, and I had a fever.

The local newspaper met us with cameras. Putting on a smile, I was interviewed and photographed with the group. "Cheryl and Troops on Trek," the headline later read, followed by an upbeat account of our undertaking. Fortunately, after a two-day rest I did feel more like the energetic trekker portrayed in the article. By the time we left, we were joined by another woman, Kris, off from college for the summer.

We headed into Nevada where the terrain was quiet desert rimmed by mountains. The highway we walked along is known as the loneliest road in America. The walking was good, and we enjoyed the occasional people who stopped to talk. We were invited by one couple who passed by to visit their small community just off the highway up ahead. We accepted and stayed for two days. One of the residents, a man named Bob, joined us when we departed and became a permanent member of our group.

At the end of miles of dusty roads, I always looked forward to my evening sponge bath. Once in a while we passed a gas station where it was possible to clean up in a bathroom with running water. (Soap and a washcloth were two of the basics I always carried in my daypack.) Finding a store with frozen yogurt was a major event. Even in the vast stretches of desert we were occasionally spotted by a news crew who would want to film and interview us, though most days were passed in alternating periods of quiet contemplation and talks with curious passersby.

Many times on the road we encountered wonderful synchronicities that I like to think of as demonstrations of grace. On one occasion, for instance, when I was driving the car, I pulled to the side of the road to set up for lunch and discovered an oversight by the food crew—we were out of supplies. It might have been a hundred miles or more before I could get to a store; there was no way I could be back with food for lunch.

While I was pondering what to do, a car pulled over and a man got out, asking what the sign on the car was all about. As I told him about our walk, he became very excited and asked if he could donate some money. After I explained our policy, he said, "Well, I have some bags of apples and some cheese in the car. Can I give you that?" So, on a lightly traveled road in the middle of nowhere, lunch came to us.

All along the way we met people—behind counters at the grocery store, at the post office, or along the road—who were interested in and enthusiastic about our walk for peace. Once, when a preacher drove by with a car full of kids on his way home from an outing, he stopped and invited us to his church for dinner and hospitality. His town was a three-day walk away. By the time we arrived, he had arranged a meeting for us to talk about our walk.

On another day we woke up to snow and walked against hail that fell in small pieces. That evening a farmer and his wife drove up and spoke with us for quite a while. Later that night the farmer came back with his sixteen-year-old son, and Andy and I sat up with them, huddling in the cold, and talked for hours. The fact that the farmer was willing to bring his son back in the cold and the dark made me realize how little opportunity many of us have to engage in open and meaningful dialogue. When they left I realized I was frozen to the bone and crawled into my sleeping bag wearing three pairs of socks, thermal underwear, sweat suit, shirt, and jacket.

When we reached the snowy peak of a mountain, we decided to

shuttle to a campground twenty miles away for a respite. After a two-day rest the sun came up on a beautiful morning, and we prepared to set out again. I left early, feeling fresh and invigorated.

At the top of the first hill I looked back in time to see the trailer with the outhouse attached rolling backward on a small incline. Someone had taken the wooden blocks from the wheels before attaching the trailer to the car. As I watched, the outhouse fell off and the door flew open, ejecting John, momentarily airborne, with pants at half-mast and feet flailing. Both John and the outhouse landed safely.

By the time we got to Colorado, several different people en route to New York had stopped to talk with us about a big peace rally to take place there on June 12. With only a few days left, we decided to temporarily halt our walk and, with the exception of A. Z., who opted to stay with the support vehicle, we all hitchhiked to New York. Our friends Ann and John Rush drove by on their way to the rally and spotted us on the road. After a happy reunion they took two members of our group with them.

Later, a large truck stopped and offered to take three of the remaining five of us. Andy and I sent the rest of the group off. The truck pulled out onto the highway and then back onto the shoulder again, the driver motioning to Andy and me. We ran up and the driver said, "Get in!" We squeezed into the sleeper area with the rest of the group.

Everyone enjoyed the friendly trucker. When he had taken us as far as he could, he radioed ahead to a truck stop, auctioning off five peace marchers to the next trucker who wanted some lively companionship. After that we went from pickup truck to van to Scout Ranger, managing to stay together all the way to Chicago. The only place we stopped was in Lincoln, Nebraska, to tour the state capital.

Between rides we encountered two difficult situations. We had slept by the side of the road on the first night, with one person at a time staying awake in rounds to keep watch. Sometime after midnight Andy was on watch, and I woke up when I heard him being hassled by two drunk men. The tension was high and I was frightened. Andy stayed cool and diffused their energy, talking to them quietly until they staggered off. Shortly afterward we were picked up by a man and his two-year-old daughter.

The next night a trucker dropped us off at a rest area just south of Chicago. Around midnight a patrolman came by and found us asleep in the short grass near the picnic area. Fondling his nightstick menacingly, he hurled angry words at us, aimed especially at the two long-haired young men in our group. He seemed to be daring us to give him an excuse to vent his fury. It was terrifying to be woken up to such intimidation. I was never more proud of the way the young men demonstrated our peaceful intention—remaining calm and keeping their wits about them.

We were finally given permission to leave amid the officer's angry threats. We walked several miles in the dark before we found a grassy protected area, where we all fell asleep exhausted.

In the morning we caught a bus to Chicago and rented a small car to drive the remaining eight hundred miles to New York. Our vests attracted a lot of attention. People stopped to talk to us all over Chicago, including a surprising number who were going to the event in New York.

With a million people gathering for the rally, we thought it incredible that we found Jeff and John—the two who had driven with Ann and John—standing on a street corner. We all headed for Central Park, where a section had been set aside for camping.

By now it was midnight. Loud bands were playing, and it looked like the party was just beginning. Andy and I walked through the park a long distance from the designated area and noise, arranging our bedrolls behind some bushes. We were awakened in the morning by angry voices quarreling over a drug deal that wasn't going well, only feet away from our barely concealed sleeping quarters. The air was tense with threatened violence. We hardly dared breathe until they were gone.

The rally that day was exciting, with several streets blocked off to cars. I'd never seen such a large and friendly crowd. We met and talked to people, had our pictures taken many times, ran into other members of our group, and even saw Ann and John. Five thousand policemen had been employed in case of violence, but the day remained peaceful and cheerful. Several times Andy and I met up with a Franciscan monk who hugged and kissed us as though we were treasured old friends. That night we crawled exhausted into our sleeping bags under some tree boughs and slept tensely in the rain.

In the morning the rain got heavier. We connected with our group at a prearranged meeting place, most of us frozen to the bone, and found a coffee shop with a pancake special. Kris's parents had sent her enough money to rent a car for the trip back to Colorado. Besides the fact that there were now seven of us, the idea of being crowded into another small car with loud music blaring for days was not appealing to Andy and me. We opted to go it alone. We bid the group good-bye and boarded a train to Newark, New Jersey, figuring to hitchhike from there.

When we got off the train, we found ourselves in a poor black neighborhood. We stopped to ask directions from a group of frowning, tough-looking young men. They stared at us hard before answering, and then one of them said, "What are you guys doin'?" We told them about our walk across the country as they scowled at us, and then they told us how to get to the freeway entrance. As we started to walk away, one of them yelled, "Hey!" With some apprehension we turned back. He said, "Oughta be more people like you!"

Before we got to the freeway, we were called over by a man washing cars behind a chain-link fence, by two street cleaners, and by some kids walking by. All of them were interested in what we were doing; the street cleaners engaged us in an earnest conversation about their experiences. As we approached the freeway entrance, a white man pulled his car over and threw open the passenger door, saying, "Get in here before you get killed! Don't you know this is a dangerous neighborhood?"

From there we went from truck to truck all day and through most of the night. In the morning we got a ride to the west side of St. Louis and walked to a shopping center for lunch. As we got back to the road we heard sirens going off. Our next ride informed us that there was a tornado warning, and we were in an area that was routinely hit. He dropped us off and the rain started. We were picked up just as the blackened sky really let loose and then dropped off at a gas station where we could stay dry under the eaves. After an hour we were offered a ride by a couple in a pickup truck (we hopped into the open back); we were barely breathing when the truck stopped 250 miles later. The driver had been drinking steadily. Exhausted, we found a dry field and spent the night.

After a breakfast of raw oats soaked in reconstituted powdered milk, we walked to a truck stop where I washed my hair and took a sponge bath before setting out again. It took us most of the day to get to Topeka, just sixty miles away. We started walking the six miles to the next highway and were picked up by a cab driver who was going that way and offered us a free ride. On the highway we were picked up by a doctor and his wife who fussed over us as though we were kids. We walked a couple of miles after they dropped us off and then slept in a beautiful field lit up with fireflies.

We got several short rides with congenial people in the morning, including a chain-smoking man in his thirties who called himself a pacifist and talked nonstop. He drove us thirty miles past his own destination to get us to a "good hitching place." From there we were picked up by a man whose sentences were peppered with profanity as he expressed his philosophy of how much the world would benefit if kids were routinely disciplined with a belt. He even told us he had accidentally broken his wife's jaw for interrupting him when he had been disciplining their son when he was two. Then he drove us to his house to pick up his wife so she could meet us and ride along while he took us to the next town. (It was forty-five miles away and he didn't want us to get stranded on the road.) His wife was lovely. We also met his kids and nephews and nieces, all delightful young people.

From town we were picked up by a young man whose wife was pregnant with their first child. His truck smelled foul with the carcasses of dead cows. The cows were used for dog food. He related stories about the slaughterhouse, including one that explained his broken arm: a cow had retained enough life to kick him when he had started to chop it up, thinking it was dead.

By nightfall we stood at the side of the road trying to absorb all of the day's experiences. Our nerves were shattered, but it gave us something to think about. We had been picked up by a varied assortment of curious individuals. Most of them were people we never would have associated with, and yet nearly all had gone out of their way to be kind to us.

The sky was black and rain imminent—and there were no trees or other shelter around. Within a short time we were picked up by Dale, who drove us several hours through the night. He had been heading north to Denver but decided to go west so he could take us all the way to Pueblo. He spent the night talking about his twenty-seven years in the army. He told how he enjoyed "roughing up" recruits, "for their own good, of course," and recounted war stories from Vietnam.

It was after midnight when we stumbled out of the jeep and, in physical and emotional exhaustion, half walked and half slipped down the hill off the highway. We bedded down behind some bushes, pulling a poncho over our sleeping bags and sleeping fitfully in the rain.

In the morning we walked three miles to a restaurant to clean up and have breakfast. We felt dirty and drained. We were within a day or two of reaching the group, but we needed time to unwind from our road experiences. We wired home for money from a fund we had set aside and found a motel with a kitchenette.

Two days later we were picked up by Richard Polese and his daughter, Tamsin, who had come to spend a couple of weeks with us on our cross-country adventure. In our absence another friend, Barbara, had joined the walk and would be with us for several weeks. It was a warm homecoming.

Whirlwind days followed as we met more people and went through more towns. We were hosted at potlucks, met by reporters, and invited to speak at various groups and churches, with contacts often being set up for us down the road.

It was into July and getting very hot. We were still picking up aluminum cans along the roads and once, when a trucker had stopped to talk with us, he got on his radio and let other truckers know what we were doing. For the rest of the day when trucks went by the drivers would throw cans out the window and flash peace signs with their fingers. Proceeds from the cans were especially welcome in the heat, when official campgrounds afforded us a cool swimming pool to jump into at the end of the day. Such cooling relief was a welcome respite.

PARTING WAYS

The weather got hotter, and during the long, warm days I worried about Cindy, who was having a difficult pregnancy. I spent most evenings knitting or cutting out patterns for baby clothes. Andy had been restless and jittery since we returned from New York. More and more often the two of us would hike into the surrounding hills in the evenings and sleep on a bluff, where we talked of our dreams and slept in each other's arms.

I knew that Andy was getting anxious to return to work; he kept in touch with his partner by phone. On July 22, as I was walking along the road, he drove by in the support vehicle and picked me up on his way into town to make his routine weekly call to the office. I was at the library when he came in excitedly. His partner had been trying to reach him, he said, so that he could come back and do some troubleshooting on a project. A ticket had already been booked for him on a flight to Salt Lake City, and he had to reach the Wichita airport, sixty miles away, in three hours.

We were driving to the trailer so he could pack a small bag when a tire blew out. We had one of those temporary spares buried under piles of gear, but time was short. I told him to leave—he'd have a better chance to make his plane if he hitched a ride. He jumped out and had gone just a few yards down the road when a car came by. He stuck out his thumb and it pulled over. He ran after it, and as he climbed in he shouted back, "Good-bye!"

It was several days and two phone calls later before I realized that Andy wasn't coming back. Not just to the walk, but to me. It had never occurred to me that we wouldn't always be together, but somehow, unbeknownst to me, the relationship had come to an end. The devastation that set in was so vast that all I could do was push the pain down so it wouldn't overwhelm me.

Nothing seemed real. I had never felt closer to Andy than I did on those recent nights we had spent together up on the bluffs. He had to have known what he was planning, and yet instead of preparing me he held me in his arms and pretended. How much of our lives together had been a lie? If something that I'd trusted with my whole heart wasn't true, then I no longer knew anything. How could I ever know what was true again? I had felt so close to him that I wasn't always sure where I ended and he began. A part of myself felt ripped away. It was just too difficult to go on. I left the walk a few weeks later to be with Cindy and to try to make sense of what had happened.

The rest of the group continued on, and in September I flew back to rejoin them. We arrived in Washington D.C. six months after our departure from San Francisco. It was October and getting very cold. We acquired a permit to hold a vigil in front of the White House for thirty-six hours, and there we were joined again by well-wishers and friends. After the vigil a service was held for us at a nearby church, where we bid one another good-bye. The walk had come to an end, and so had my marriage.

How had my life gotten so off-kilter? I had been sure that Andy and I would be partners for life. Sometimes I wished he had died so I wouldn't feel so abandoned and betrayed. Then I hated myself for such thoughts. On the outside I defended him. It wasn't his fault. I should have been more aware or more sensitive. How could I not have known that something was wrong?

Months later Andy was admitted to a Veteran's hospital for post-traumatic stress relating back almost twenty years to his experiences in Vietnam. In retrospect I could see how our road experiences might have opened up old wounds. Still, how could anything explain his adamant refusal to see or talk to me? My fears and guilt were monsters by night, following me like shadows during the day.

A. Z., as surprised as anyone by Andy's departure, came to spend Christmas with me. He never left, and his attention turned romantic. He was my best friend and he loved me. In time I transferred my feelings from the first Andy to the second, even calling A. Z. by his real name, Andy. That part of the transition was easy. Eventually we flew to Hawaii to exchange vows.

Designing our life together now, the second Andy and I bought an almond orchard in California and set out to build a retreat center. For a year we lived in a little trailer. We drew up the plans for our house and built it ourselves. In the beginning it was a peaceful existence. The trailer was set back from the road on which barely a half-dozen cars went by in the course of a day. At nightfall, invisible behind the trees, we bathed in a plastic children's swimming pool in water that had been warmed by the sun. In a simple way it was idyllic.

Hard work, punctuated with laughter and tears, went into the building of our home. It was an incredible feeling to watch it rise up out of our own labor. But despite how well things seemed to be going outwardly, part of me had disengaged from life. Just beneath the surface lay heaps of guilt and loss that I had no words for. The pain inside of me was so great that it had to be felt by Andy who, in his frustration, lashed out in ways that made me feel more and more lost and humiliated. I felt like a jackhammer was pounding me into the ground, and I receded further and further away.

After the house was finished I kept very busy. I took a hatha yoga teacher's training course in the Bahamas and went back to school to finish my degree in psychology. Andy and I traveled and gave presentations together. We organized and led retreats. For five years we struggled to make it work. Tension built easily between us and stress took its toll.

As time went on I became more and more tired. With no forewarning drowsiness, I could drop instantly into sleep any time of day.

When I woke up in the car one afternoon, by myself, going seventy miles an hour into a field beside the highway, I had to admit that something was wrong. There were plenty of other warning signs. I knew that I couldn't hold up under the constant strain. "This has to stop. It's killing me," I told Andy at a time when the tension between us was explosive. I didn't know it yet, but cancer had taken hold. When he wouldn't agree to come to joint counseling with me I knew that I could no longer stay.

I had no strength left. In exhaustion and defeat I packed and left the house we had built together. Everything that had been familiar and certain was in the process of disintegration. I was like the caterpillar that has wrapped itself in a tight cocoon, unable to see beyond the protective layers I had built around myself. I had no vision for the future, and the present was blanketed in darkness.

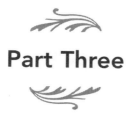

Part Three

Reengaging Life

16

Surviving the Dark Night

Not everything that is faced can be changed,
but nothing can be changed until it is faced.

JAMES BALDWIN

With senses dimmed, I was catapulted into the proverbial dark night of the soul. The temptation toward despair and hopelessness was seeping in. Self-destruction seemed a real danger.

As I experienced my own cycle of despair, I felt like an individual representation of what was happening on a much larger scale in the world. Just as individuals falling into desperation use various subtle and not so subtle means to self-destruct, I could see the same dynamic reflected collectively. Humanity was racing toward mass destruction of various life forms, threatening the planet that supported our very existence. The things that were happening to me on a personal level were happening on all levels during this period of great transition. Cancer as a concept was pervasive—and continues to be.

DARKNESS OR TRANSFORMATION

No matter how isolated I felt at times, I was part of the whole. On some level I realized that each of us is making a choice as to whether we are willing to mature and grow from a physical and emotional—or ego—perspective to a more spiritual one. It is a journey that can feel like death and loss; the outcome, personally and globally, is in our hands. We have an opportunity to embrace the inner journey, to recognize the power of tuning in to our own higher natures, and to step into creative and fulfilling lives.

The challenges that come to us can be a calling to open our field of vision to new directions. Yet when things that are familiar or taken for granted begin to disintegrate, it is tempting to give up or turn to despair. The darkness that descends can lead to self-destruction, but it can also be a catalyst for transformation to a higher order. It can push us, if we're willing, through the barriers of unconsciousness, dissipating the terrors and fears that lie hidden. We cannot heal what we continue to hide away.

In Greek the word for *soul* is also the word for *butterfly*. In order to take wing the butterfly must first break out of the chrysalis that has created the context for transformation to take place. The struggle is intense and takes every bit of strength that the emerging butterfly has. Out of compassion we might hasten to aid the butterfly in its journey to freedom, but in so doing we would cripple the butterfly for life. It is only through the butterfly's own effort of pushing itself through the tiny opening in the chrysalis that blood is forced into its wings, allowing it to fly.

And so it is in the soul's journey. We have to push ourselves through the tiny opening of our spiritual awakening toward the light of freedom. Whether we're dealing with an illness or some other condition or situation in life, we must take responsibility for our own healing. Doctors and other resources can help to stabilize and control physical symptoms or life circumstances, but healing, if it is to be permanent, is a condition of learning and growing on our part.

THE SACRED JOURNEY

The profound healing I'm referring to takes place on a soul level and may or may not mean staying in the body. It is a sacred journey into a realm that can only be perceived by the eyes of the higher nature.

While there is no way to scientifically measure or validate the existence of a higher nature, we can know it through an awakening within. It is the altruistic inner voice that calls us to recognize the reigning power of love, the greatest power for healing and transforming that which is out of harmony, both within us and in our world.

The journey entails breaking through constricting and limiting belief systems, including our identification with the body that we inhabit. The body is seen by the higher nature as a vehicle we are using in this lifetime, a suit of clothes, rather than as who or what we are. We are the spark that animates the body, and that spark goes on without beginning or end.

When we see ourselves from the perspective of ongoing spirit, we have less attachment to the survival of our bodies; paradoxically, as we get our lives into harmony with universal love, we have more energy available to heal our bodies. When we embark on this spiritual journey, however, whether we heal our bodies or make the transition and let our bodies go is not what matters. What matters is how we use the life we are given in this very moment.

Spiritual healing comes with a profound sense of inner peace and well-being. Physical healing often follows, although in the bigger picture the soul follows its calling and continues its journey on either side of life. We heal at an unconscious level all the time, but when we enter into a conscious and participatory journey we tap into extraordinary possibilities.

Without energy our physical bodies would be inanimate and lifeless. From our first breath our physical bodies are infused with energy from the nurturing forces around us such as air, water, food, and warmth. An outer balance can be reached by following the rules of physical health: breathing in fresh air, drinking pure water, eating a nourishing diet, and getting plenty of exercise, sunshine, and rest. An inner balance can be attained by following the universal principles of forgiveness and compassion in our dealings with both ourselves and others. This is the journey that strengthens our connection to that universal source so that it is open and flowing.

The spiritual awareness that develops through putting the higher principles into practice is powerful not because it lifts us above physical laws and suffering, but because it helps us to live a life of positive influence and purpose. Whenever we notice beauty, for example, we increase the beauty in the world. As we heal ourselves, we help to heal everyone and everything around us. We can all be miracle makers. Few of us are called to perform miracles in the greater public eye, but we can all perform them every day, whenever we use a word of good cheer to uplift a harried grocery clerk or to encourage the efforts of a child struggling to learn something new.

Facing catastrophic illness or any other difficulty can be experienced as an invitation to embark on a sacred journey where, instead of merely scratching the surface of life, we become aware of the awesome gift that we have to create and live out lives that are purposeful, joyful, and vibrant. Few, relatively speaking, have the opportunity to perceive the preciousness of life with the same intensity that is reserved for those who have faced life-threatening challenges.

Yet today is the only day any of us can live. Yesterday is gone, and we don't know what tomorrow will bring. This is the time that we have, right now in the present moment, and it's up to us to determine how we will use it.

17

Time in the Wilderness

*Nature is painting for us, day after day, pictures of
infinite beauty if only we have eyes to see them.*

JOHN RUSKIN

Cancer brought many changes and many new experiences into my
life. While I was living in my little studio about a year after my diagnosis, my friend Jeff Blom contacted me about leading two wilderness canoe retreats in the summer. A veteran wilderness expert,
Larry Miner, would accompany us and handle the logistics along
with Jeff. I would be responsible for planning the food and leading
group discussions focused on Peace Pilgrim and her steps toward
inner peace.

The trip would take us down the Green River in Utah. As Larry
described it, "The river is calm, no rapids, and winds its way through
deep, sheer red canyon walls. The weather should be sunny and hot
with the possibility of showers. The water offers good swimming and
a pleasant current that does most of the work. The side canyons make
for fun exploring and camping."

The last thing Peace had asked me to do before she died was to
help her organize a retreat. Now this invitation would give me an
opportunity to complete that intention. She was no longer with us in
the flesh, but I felt she would accompany us in spirit. I was feeling
good, and even if the future was uncertain it seemed safe to assume I'd

be around long enough to lead the retreats. I accepted Jeff's invitation with enthusiasm.

I arrived a day early in Moab, Utah, the starting point for our journey, to meet with Jeff and Larry. I immediately fell in love with the colorful little town. The lively streets buzzed with friendly people going in and out of quaint shops and museums. And from just about anywhere you could look out to the red rocky cliffs that surrounded the town like timeless ancient guardians. The spellbinding horizons pulled the strings of ancient collective memories that reside somewhere inside me.

On the morning of departure, participants gathered at the outfitter's for orientation. As we all swapped introductions we were greeted by the proprietor, a man named Tex. Tex was a wiry, exuberant character who could have stepped out of an old Western novel. He told stories with gusto and humor while warning us of the serious importance of cooperating with one another and with nature as we ventured out onto the river. We would have no contact with civilization until we were picked up by jet boat seven days hence.

Things turned chaotic as the group's gear piled up to be loaded onto the old bus that would drive us to the river. A trailer attached to the bus was stacked with the six canoes that would carry us through our adventure. At Larry's direction to "get things moving," all the food I had so painstakingly organized was pulled out of bags and loaded helter-skelter into a collection of coolers and bins. Twelve virtual strangers climbed aboard and started to get acquainted on the drive to the river's edge.

At the departure point we met our first challenge—how to steer a canoe. I had never even been in a canoe before, and neither had at least half of the group. Larry was our instructor. Before we launched he demonstrated the simple techniques we would need to know and matched one skilled (however slightly) with one unskilled partner in each canoe. When we pushed out from shore, we resembled a school of minnows, weaving from one side of the river to the other as we attempted to maneuver downstream.

We needed to cover a minimum of twenty miles a day in order to reach the confluence of the Green and Colorado Rivers, our pickup point, on the scheduled day. We made it to our first destination with several weary participants, of which I was certainly one. The river might have done most of the work, but there was plenty left over for us.

Reaching camp didn't mean the work was over. It was a job to get all the canoes tied securely and the gear unloaded up steep muddy embankments. We learned early on to form lines and pass gear along. Once the unloading was done, the food crew, which rotated daily, set up the kitchen. The rest of the group scouted out the best places to set up tents or ground cloths, each person claiming a space that would be home for the night.

Larry and Jeff formed the latrine crew, a challenge they admirably rose to. The toilet, a rectangular metal ammo can lined with large disposable plastic bags, was positioned out of sight behind trees. A standard toilet seat fit onto the ammo can for comfort, and toilet paper was available inside a plastic bag. Deluxe accommodations for roughing it, and often with a lovely view of the river.

The canyon lands speak volumes in silence. It is a land of cliffs, canyons, arches, spires, and mesas carved by water and time. Formations are layered in white sandstone, with layers of silt and mud deposits that range in color from gold and brown to bright red orange. In this beautiful but seemingly inhospitable and arid country, evidence of the passage of ancient peoples is carved into the protected faces of cliffs where petroglyphs representing animals, hand- and footprints, rivers or snakes, and unique human figures titillate the imagination.

Rock structures for shelter or food storage were built into cliffs that, while sometimes accessible, at other times appear impossible to reach. The magic of the place and its history are awesome. No matter how many times I return to that river, it is always an excursion into the past where present realities and modernization fade into temporary oblivion.

It can also be a harsh environment. Several days into the first trip we glided down the brown river watching warily as storm clouds formed over the surrounding cliffs. The day darkened. We had been looking for a place to tie in, but there had been only sheer cliffs for some miles. A fierce head wind came up, further straining our progress as we steered into it.

With a loud crack the clouds burst into a downpour of flying pellets that pounded the canoes with the fury of angry little fists. Lightning added its deadly threat as we struggled to head the six canoes toward a sandbar that had come into view. As the last canoe was hauled onto solid ground, we gave a brief sigh of relief, scrambling to pull out ponchos and ground cloths to cover ourselves and what gear we could.

I managed to get into a poncho and sank to the ground, exhausted. Shivers were taking over my body and I just gave in to them. Several people gathered around, pushing my arms into a warm coat and pulling a blanket around me. We grouped into a huddle until the storm blew over and the warm sun emerged.

When the rain stopped we looked around in amazement at newly formed waterfalls that were cascading down rocky cliffs in every direction. Then the sky turned into a canvas of pastel hues as invisible fingers painted a full double rainbow over the horizon. I had never seen such a dramatic contrast as this sudden shift from ferocious storm to spectacular painting.

We watched in quiet reverence for some time before loading ourselves back into the canoes to find a more secure beach to camp on for the night. Most of us were too tired to explore after dinner, so we had an early group meeting and then separated. Most of us wanted only to relax on the white sandy beach that, like our gear, was already dried by the afternoon sun.

I lay on my back on the ground cloth I had spread out earlier and drifted, partly asleep and partly aware of the subdued voices around me in the dimming light. I heard a flapping sound near my head and felt a plop on my chest, but I was too relaxed and too far away to open my eyes. I heard Jeff's voice in the distance: "Did you see that? A dove landed on the sand and hopped on Cheryl's chest!" A dove, the symbol of peace. A sign from Peace? *Yes, you are with us in spirit,* I thought, as I slipped into a deep sleep.

In the morning we had to set out early to reach the pickup point at the confluence of the rivers by noon. My body was still somewhat fragile and had been strained by the unfamiliar stress of living outdoors and rowing against wind and rain. The red rocks went by in a blur. It was a thrill to pull up on the last shore of the trip where the jet boat would pick us up. The sky was overcast again and threatening rain. The boat came. So did the rain.

Wet cold blew over us in a rush as the boat sped along. It would take us four hours to get up the river to where the bus waited to take us into town. I curled up on the floor wrapped in my sleeping bag and continued to shiver. Jeff opened his bag and added it to the bulk already covering me.

We were scheduled to take the next group out in the morning; this meant I would need to do my laundry and all the food shopping for the next group that night. There was no way I could do it. My energy was drained. If I could have just one day to check into a motel and sleep, I thought I might be OK. I called Jeff over and asked him to arrange with Larry to meet the group without me in the morning and spend the day hiking in Arches National Park just outside town. They could check with the outfitter to see if we could put in the day after tomorrow at a point half the distance of what we'd covered this time. Jeff made the arrangements.

The storm clouds looked much friendlier from my motel window after a good night's sleep. By evening when the group met for dinner, I found out that they'd spent much of the day telling stories underneath a rocky cliff, protected from the rain. The weather certainly wouldn't have provided a good introduction to the river. But the next morning dawned under clear blue skies. This time we put in at Mineral Bottom, only fifty-three miles from the confluence, with six days to make the trip.

The adventure began with a bus ride to the new departure point. A few miles before reaching the river we had to follow steep switchbacks down a canyon wall. Most of us got out at the steepest point of the grade and walked a mile or so while the bus waited on top for a few minutes to give us a head start. At the bottom where the grade leveled off, we waited for the bus to creep down the narrow curves and pick us up again.

This was the same river I had just been on, but the trip was very different this time. With fewer miles to cover each day we were able to explore many side canyons and Anasazi ruins. The miles of paddling were broken with long breaks to swim and enjoy the cooling river. We even indulged in mud baths that were surely equal to what can be experienced in a luxury spa.

Whenever we managed to camp on a flat sandy surface, I would lead yoga at dawn, followed by our usual morning meditations. The days were warm, sometimes hot, but the river offered relief from the heat. There were no more rains.

The kitchen became the natural gathering place at the end of the day with many more helpers than the two whose turn it might officially be. The meals I'd planned were simple, all vegetarian, and yet they were received as feasts as the fresh air and exercise whetted our appetites.

After dinner we would gather to listen to stories about Peace and to add our own. Lively debates drifted into quiet musings as the sun settled into the horizon. The evening often ended in song. Words and music seemed to carry greater impact in this natural setting; many of us reached deep inner recesses as we explored our own beings and the nature of life.

As I made my way down the river for the second time, the external trappings of modern life withdrew further and further, and the stillness that often gets lost in the midst of frantic schedules and obligations began to permeate both inner and outer realms. My body fell into a rhythm as I dipped my oar into the water and pulled it through. It became less a chore and more a joining with the flow as my arms found their strength and guided the canoe with almost effortless ease.

Unbridled wilderness extended in every direction. I could feel the patterns of my habitual thinking recede while the intuitive and more primitive parts of my mind edged forward and tuned in to the esoteric language of nature.

The most difficult adjustments on such trips, I learned, usually come during the first two days out as participants learn to maneuver canoes, lug heavy loads up and down steep paths, bathe in muddy water, and attempt to keep sand from blowing into their food. There were times in the first few days when I'm sure some individuals would have turned back if they could. But then something almost imperceptible would start to happen: an expanding of awareness as the finite "me" in each of us cracked open in varying degrees, allowing a grander view into our vast potential and making connection with the infinite "I am."

For many of us, living outdoors rekindled an intrinsic connection with the Earth that manifested in increased energy and vitality—despite the exposure to the elements and added expenditures of energy. The Earth soaked up energy from the sun by day and radiated it back into the environment by night, revitalizing our bodies as we rested unsheltered under star-studded skies.

By the time we passed Turtle Rock on the second trip, marking our merger into the confluence of the Green and Colorado Rivers and signaling the end of the journey, I had undergone a physical transformation. Unlike the previous week when I had come off the river exhausted, my body now felt invincible. Without a doubt, I had entered a new level in my healing.

For the next four years I was drawn back to lead retreats down the Green River. Living outdoors without the usual comforts and conveniences brought out both weaknesses and strengths in the various participants as we went along. And in varying degrees, the river brought out the poet, the writer, the artist, the philosopher, or the explorer in each of us. For some, the experience was life changing. For others, it provided at least a time-out from the usual structures and routines of everyday life.

After hot sunny days we always found relief in the cooling evening temperatures. Fifteen strangers bathed under brilliant night stars, shared parts of our innermost selves, bonded and became intimate friends. I watched again and again during various retreats how resistance and judgment gave way to tolerance, and then acceptance and finally respect, among individuals who under ordinary circumstances might not have given themselves an opportunity to know one another.

Here on the river, this neutral place outside of our usual existence, we could examine Peace's steps toward inner peace and view with some perspective where we were in our own lives. During Peace's "spiritual growing up" years, she had wrestled with what many of us were currently experiencing as the duality in ourselves—the struggle between the higher nature, or conscience, and the lower nature, or ego. To my mind there was something mysteriously powerful about these discussions in the wilderness. Our rational minds, with their limited perspective, seemed to have room to stretch beyond the boundaries we ordinarily set for ourselves.

Our last overnight stop on each of the retreats was on the lip of an extraordinary canyon that I called "the Garden of the Gods" because of the multitude of faces carved by nature into the surrounding rock walls. As we maneuvered our way along the constantly changing bank of the river (it changed not only from week to week, but also dramatically from year to year), I kept a lookout for the landmark I knew I couldn't miss—the monolith rock monkey on a throne that would come into view on the right as we rounded the bend before Jasper Canyon. It was our cue for the lead canoe to cut across the current and search out the best access to the upper ledge, on which we would camp. We often reached the site a day early so we could spend an extra day relaxing and enjoying the bountiful treasures of this particular area.

One of the attractions was an Anasazi ruin partway up a rock wall that could be seen from the ground. The more adventurous would climb up to an adjacent cliff for a closer look. I had climbed up one day and was on my way down when a young woman above me lost her balance as the rock she grabbed gave way.

I watched as she somersaulted backward, righting herself as she catapulted past me. My eyes captured in slow motion the calm, focused look on her face. There wasn't a sound as the twelve people on the ground and the two of us on the cliff held her in our eyes. She landed on her feet like a ballerina, bent her knees gracefully, and straightened into a standing position. "I'm fine," she said in a calm voice before taking in, as we all did, her extraordinary fall.

She had confided to the group earlier that she had joined this retreat in an effort to recover her courage and sense of personal safety. Now here she stood without so much as a sprained ankle. It was a turning point for her, and a gift for those of us who had witnessed it.

Other intrepid explorers on one of the early retreats caused us to venture deep into Jasper Canyon and discover yet another wonder to add to our desert odyssey. The hike started past the ruins, following the canyon floor where deep rust-colored jasper rocks began to mingle with turquoise and various colored hues. After scrambling around huge boulders for several minutes and crossing a marblelike ballroom floor of flat rock, we rounded the last bend, walking into an exquisitely sculptured natural amphitheater.

The first time I saw it, I was startled by the garden of green vegetation in this rocky desert terrain. Drops spattered into the puddles of water dotting the patches of greenery and drew our attention to water sprinkling down in a thin waterfall from a natural spring out of view some hundred feet up. Swarms of small frogs leapt at our feet on our first visit. We could lie under the falling drops with sunglasses on to protect our eyes and follow the path of individual droplets that fell like wriggling blobs of Jell-O.

We discovered a strange phenomenon in this magical place. If we stood just outside the range of falling drops, the water would slowly move until it reached and then covered us where we stood. It was a mystery we were thrilled to experience again and again.

On my final excursion leading a group down the Green River, we asked out loud to the group and silently to ourselves the age-old questions, "Who am I?" and "What is my purpose in life?" Here, we had a unique perspective, away from the usual distractions.

A young man, Mike, expressed the doubts he had been experiencing. He had come to this retreat in search of some inner confirmation of his faith and of his direction in life. He told us about his endeavors as a seminary student and spoke of a hospital where he worked with prisoners. He had been touched by the calm and peaceful demeanor of a young black man, strapped to his bed, who'd taught him a beautiful hymn, which Mike now taught to us: *Surely goodness and kindness will follow me, all the days, all the days of my life.*

We hiked as a group into the canyon to explore the natural amphitheater, the crown jewel of this wilderness experience. I led the group near the waterfall to demonstrate the unexplainable phenomenon of how the water moved toward us when we stood near it. I said it would happen, holding my breath and wondering if it really would—or was it some magic spell that had disappeared? We stood around until faces lit up in amazement and laughter as the water moved, covering individuals in a light shower. Mike stood off to one side, holding his arms out, watching as the water sprayed one after another of us—but not him.

"Let's sing Mike's song," I called out to the group, asking him to lead. His deep, rich voice began: *Surely goodness and kindness will follow me, all the days, all the days of my life.* His eyes were closed as he sang the words, but they opened, startled, as the water covered him in a refreshing shower.

18

Embracing the Possibilities

All things are possible until they are proved impossible—
and even then the impossible may only be so as of now.
PEARL S. BUCK

Several years had passed since my diagnosis of cancer had brought a deepening awareness of the potential in each new day. Any life-shaking event can bring a new perspective from which to examine the various aspects of our lives. If we choose to allow it, even seeming tragedies can bring incredible growth.

Peace once said that 98 percent of all illness is psychologically induced. Research confirms the role that emotions and unrelenting stress can play in the development of pathology. In that sense, the body can be a barometer for our well-being. When we live out of integrity with our beliefs, or ignore aspects of our lives that need attention, or become overwhelmed by stress, we have an inner guidance system that speaks through the body. If we address only the symptoms and not the message, our inner guidance will keep finding ways to communicate; thus, a condition may reappear or a new one take its place.

Dreams are another way in which the mind processes various events in our lives and works on solutions to a problem, communicating messages through the language of metaphor. Not every dream is important to analyze, but when a dream elicits a strong emotional response or carries a sense of importance, there is almost always something of value to be learned from looking at it.

Five years after my diagnosis I had a dream that seemed insignificant in content, but as I recalled it upon awakening I felt very emotional. I couldn't shake the feeling. When I went walking in the hills surrounding my house that afternoon, tears rolled down my cheeks. It was puzzling because I couldn't identify any reason for the tears. The feelings were simply coming up as a result of that dream.

In the wonderful way of synchronicity, I attended a workshop on dreams the next day taught by my friend Randal Churchill. When Randal asked if anyone had a recent dream they'd like to work on, my hand popped up before I was consciously aware of even thinking about volunteering. Randal was demonstrating a process he had developed called Hypnotic Dreamwork, in which the object is not to analyze or interpret a dream, but to experience the dream by becoming different parts of it, thus getting the meaning on a deep and personal level.

Sitting in a chair facing Randal in front of the class, I explained that my dream didn't seem important but the details were very vivid. Randal asked me to close my eyes and describe the dream as though it were happening in the present:

I'm deciding to get on a bus to take an early-morning ride around the city, and I have a little dog with me. After a while I notice that the bus isn't moving, and I suddenly realize that I need to be home by nine o'clock for an appointment. I also notice now that the bus seems much roomier inside. It's more like a train, with people lounging around.

I go up to ask the bus driver what time the bus is going to be back to the stop where I got on, and he says, "The bus will be back there around nine o'clock." I sit back down and look at my watch. It's about a quarter to nine. I think, Well, this bus doesn't look like it's going to move. Then I realize, Oh my gosh! Does he mean nine o'clock tonight?

I go up again and say, "Excuse me, but did you mean nine o'clock this evening?" He says, "Well, sure." I ask if there are any other buses

I can take or any other way I can get home. He starts to tell me, but his plan sounds really complicated. Then he says, "Why don't you just go out? There are some lovely marketplaces around here."

I step out and realize that we must have traveled some distance because this looks like Mexico. The marketplace is a food market, and the terrain is very dusty and dry. Some children are holding my little dog for me while I decide whether I'm going to stay and enjoy the marketplace or whether I've got to figure out this complicated way to get back. And then I wake up.*

Relating a dream in that way taps a person into a light hypnotic state, which I could feel myself going into. Randal then directed me into a gestalt process whereby I imagined being different parts of the dream. I started by imagining being the bus—what I as the bus looked like and where I was going. I lay down on the floor and spread my arms wide, describing myself as bigger and roomier than I'd been before—more open and lighter; not on such a hectic schedule. It was surprising to hear myself using words that described changes I had been feeling in my life. I liked being the more expanded bus.

Randal then asked me to sit down facing an empty chair. I was to be myself, walking around the marketplace and debating whether or not to go back. The empty chair represented the bus. When Randal asked if I had anything to say to the bus, intense emotion gathered in my chest. (Hypnotic states open a pathway to the subconscious mind where emotions and memories are stored.) I described feeling a lot of stress in my body and a quivering sensation. Randal pointed out that my hands were clenched into fists and encouraged me to clench them tighter to exaggerate the emotion.

The decision about whether or not to look for the way back was making me squirm. "Is that what you're tense about?" Randal asked. A date suddenly flashed into my mind. The very next day would mark

*The dream and the session in its entirety can be found in the book *Become the Dream: The Transforming Power of Hypnotic Dreamwork*, by Randal Churchill (see bibliography).

five years since my diagnosis of advanced cancer. I'd had no conscious recollection of the date, but somehow the memory surfaced from my subconscious mind. Insights began pouring in and continued to come in the days following the dream work.

Despite how diligently I had worked to keep the possibilities open, some part of my subconscious had registered the prognosis of probable death, and I had been living my life in increments ever since. I would take on small projects, work that extended for six months at a time, but nothing long-term.

The dream brought a new reality to my conscious mind: in the process of accepting the role of learning and teaching how to die well, I had become well. This marked another turning point in my healing process. I had a whole future before me. It was time to look at what direction my life was to take.

At home I turned to my journal and wrote, "I want to live passionately, that is, with spontaneity and joy. I want to fill my life with simple pleasures—walks in the woods and on white sandy beaches; new and interesting friends and relationships; a livelihood that allows me to be in charge of myself and in harmony with my purpose in life. I want to reengage life without illness or guilt."

"If my life could be exactly how I want it to be, what would it look like?" I wrote the question down in a section of my journal where I now perform a yearly exercise of envisioning my life as I would ideally like it to be. I imagined and wrote out what kind of environment I'd want to live in, the kinds of things I'd like to do for my livelihood, what I would like in the way of financial security, what my ideal relationships would be like, what I'd like to do for recreation and inspiration.

I put myself in the position of director and writer of the character who lived my life. What kind of person would I like to be? I wrote in detail my vision of every aspect of how I saw myself in the ideal. Then I released it, trusting life to bring me the perfect opportunities and challenges to guide me where I needed to go.

It's amazing to look back now, years later, on that first journal entry. So much of what seemed liked wonderful fantasies have unfolded into reality—and in many ways much more wonderful than I ever imagined.

Life, with all its wake-up calls, continues to teach me and deepen the lessons. Love is the most powerful force there is. Forgiveness opens up the closed places that keep us from giving and receiving love. Everything that comes to us comes for a reason, even though we don't always see the bigger picture. Life essentially is good. And struggles, if we're willing to learn from them, wake us up to the incredible potential within us to live meaningful lives of beauty and wonder and fulfillment.

19

Healing Stories

*To heal is to touch with love that which
we previously touched with fear.*

STEPHEN LEVINE

From birth until death we are infused with energy from the air, water, food, and sun that we take in, but there is also another kind of energy. Peace referred to it as a universal source that never runs out; she stated that without it she never would have been able to undertake her unusual calling.

She told a story about a trucker who pulled over when he saw her walking. He had heard her talk about that "endless energy" on the radio, and he wanted to tell her that he had experienced it once. "I was marooned in a town by a flood, and I got so bored that I offered to help. I got interested in getting people out and I worked without eating or sleeping and wasn't tired. But I don't have that energy anymore." Peace asked him what he was working for now and he said, "Money."

"That should be quite incidental," Peace told him. "You have that endless energy only when you're working for the good of the whole. That's the secret of it. In this world you're given as you give. Just as you cannot receive without giving, you cannot give without receiving—even the most wonderful things like health and happiness and inner peace."

The kind of energy we get from the elements brings an outer balance, which we can nurture by following the physical rules of health. This is the kind of balance or healing we can seek from doctors. But profound healing comes from an inner balance that can be reached only when our connection to that universal source is open and flowing. Negative emotions, such as resentment or guilt or vengeance, not only drain the energy we get from the elements, but also block our connection to that universal source. The practice of forgiveness and compassion opens the connection to that universal flow so that profound healing can occur.

When profound healing does come, it is with a penetrating sense of inner peace and a faith that everything is going to be all right. No matter what happens externally, we know that we are in our right place and that we have the inner resources to deal with whatever comes.

The way I experienced healing was not in one dramatic moment, but in a series of realizations amid various struggles which offered deepening insights: when I woke up and knew I could deal with death naturally; when I perceived my cancer cells as frightened young children; and when I experienced compassion moving through me where fear or bitterness had been. During each of these moments and others, I knew that something major had shifted inside. I didn't know whether I would live or die, but I knew that, whatever happened, I would be all right.

As we become attuned to a deeper inner reality, our perspective continually grows, and we begin to recognize certain universal principles. There are no accidents in the unfolding of events; in all things, there is a divine order that we can trust. Death is the final experience we all have on Earth. If it comes early in life, this may be the natural order of our life plan, or we may be being called elsewhere, or we may have agreed on some level to serve in the learning or healing of someone close to us as we make the transition. As difficult as it is to be physically separated from our loved ones, death does not remove that connection between hearts, and grief is a natural process that can lead to healing and growth.

Most of us are not consciously aware of the big picture, but we can feel and hold an inner awareness of our connection to something greater than ourselves. We know that we will all experience an eventual shedding of the physical body, and letting go of trying to control the timing frees our energies to work on healing. The "I" in each of us is that spiritual essence that animates the body and continues on in our evolution toward wholeness. We continue our soul's journey whether we heal and go on in this life or heal and pass on to the other side.

As spiritual awareness deepens, so does the understanding that we are here to learn and grow. If we understand that all things that come to us serve a purpose and hold some opportunity, then to ask for any circumstance to be removed would be a step backward. Rather than ask for our lessons to be removed, we can use prayer to ask for guidance and strength on the path ahead. Receptive silence or meditation is a powerful form of prayer in which we open ourselves to inspiration and to the profound healing that comes when we follow that inner guidance.

Inspiration comes in many ways: through receptive silence, dreams, uplifting writings, great teachers, people we know, or stories we hear. It comes through the simple example of ordinary people who touch something in us that lifts us up. The stories that follow are examples of some of the many ways in which individuals tap into that universal source of healing.

A SPIRITUAL HEALING

On one of the river retreats we were accompanied by a couple named Karen and Bob. Karen had been trained as a professional singer but had stopped singing after experiencing a painful trauma many years earlier. When we hiked as a group to the magical amphitheater on our final day, she began to tell us about the trauma she had suffered and her yearning to sing again. She had composed two songs but hadn't sung them out loud, and now she wanted to try.

An attentive audience climbed onto rock formations mottled with wind holes that resembled Swiss cheese, while Karen stood in front of us. When she first started to sing her voice was soft, but the natural acoustics of the place carried the sound, which grew stronger as her courage built. Her voice was unimaginably sweet. She finished one song and paused as we sat in silence, tears running down our faces. With a deep breath she launched into the second song, holding us spellbound.

Shortly after returning home Karen found out she had cancer. She and her husband joined us on another river retreat the following summer, and she stated with confidence that she had been physically healed. She was radiantly aglow, following her calling of using her voice to inspire others. Until her death a few years later she continued to sing, uplifting audiences with the unique quality of her voice. What she had mistaken for a physical healing had been a much deeper transformation, as she recovered her gift and purpose in this life before making her transition.

HEALING LOVE

My mother was the person who first demonstrated to me the importance of listening to our inner wisdom when she chose not to have further surgery for breast lumps more than twenty years ago, thirteen years before my cancer experience. Then several years later she went through a period during which she was experiencing bouts of fatigue. She went to Dr. Lynch for a checkup, and tests were taken that showed she had a low-thyroid condition. She was told she would need to go on a synthetic thyroid medication to gain back her normal level of energy. "For how long?" she asked, and the doctor said, "For life. I've never known this condition to get better on its own. It only gets worse."

The next day my mother was in my office, telling me what the doctor had said. She didn't want to take the medication except as a last resort, and she already had an alternative plan mapped out: she had started a tai chi class in which, among other things, she was gaining some understanding of the body's energy centers; she was renewing her practice of daily meditation for inner guidance; and she wanted me to work with her using visualization and positive suggestions.

We started getting together for weekly sessions. My tactic was to use progressive relaxation and imagery to get past the conscious mind to the subconscious—the part of the mind that runs the automatic body processes such as respiration and forms a link to our intuition or inner guidance system.

The subconscious understands and responds to images and symbols, whether real or imagined, making visualization a very powerful tool for consciously initiating positive changes. (Imagine cutting open a lemon and squeezing the juice into your mouth. An automatic response to the sour taste, when vividly imagined, produces salivation.)

Imagine that you're stepping into an inviting and peaceful white mist. Through the mist you can see a forest of tall trees stretching up toward the sky and beautiful flowering bushes growing along the edge of a path. Take in all the glowing colors turned pastel in the mist. Notice the sound of chirping birds and leaves fluttering in a gentle breeze.

The path looks inviting and you step onto it, hearing the sound of water in the distance, perhaps a waterfall or a moving stream. Everything is made softer in the mist, and you feel very safe and protected, bathed in its light. Imagine the light flooding you with protection. You can accept this light of protection into yourself, into your own inner being, the center within you where you are calm and safe. You can relax into this center, content just to be here in this moment.

You recognize this inner sanctuary, this place where you are calm and peaceful and strong. You can be with your inner self here, the real you. The outer self is what you present to the world. This inner self dwells within you, peaceful, secure, giving and receiving love. Your inner self is calm. Life from this center is joyful. You can relax into the experiences that come into your life, knowing that everything that comes provides you with the fullest opportunities for growing and learning.

You can see yourself flowing along with the experiences that come to you. As you flow you can imagine that the things that touch you are the treasures of life. Even when things don't appear to be treasures at first, as you allow yourself to have the experience you find the treasure contained therein. These treasures come in the various experiences of life, as you learn to trust yourself, to trust God, finding your strength and compassion and confidence in so many ways.

Now while in this beautiful light mist, this mystical place, feeling the peaceful tranquillity, experiencing what might feel like being held in loving compassion, imagine yourself being filled with the healing energy of love and light. Imagine that love spilling forth from you like a fountain. You can send this love in the form of light to all those who are close to you and to the whole world beyond.

From this place, now, you can get in touch with your inner discerning mind, your higher self. You can ask this inner guidance to begin to reveal certain insights regarding healing in the area of your thyroid. These insights might have to do with a certain way you're spending energy. Sometimes energy is spent on misconceptions that develop at some point, perhaps early in life, that put a negative slant on how we see ourselves or the world. Or you might have some insight about some aspect of your life that has gotten out of balance or harmony. Or perhaps this experience is giving you an opportunity to serve or give back in some way, or it might be an opportunity to appreciate the many ways in which your body is working well and serving you in your life. I'm going to be silent for a few moments while you get in touch with your inner discerning mind. (Pause.)

As insights come to you, you can begin to release and let go of old patterns or misconceptions that have held you back in any way, and move on to increasingly deeper and richer experiences of the wonder and beauty in the world. Trusting life to bring you exactly the right lessons for your learning and growth.

A part of your mind can continue with the image of radiating love and light while you ask your higher self, your inner guidance, to send you just the right inspiration for healing, balance and harmony throughout your body and your mind and your emotions and your spirit. Bring warmth and balance and harmony throughout the cells of your body. Every cell contains a memory and a map of perfect health and harmony and balance.

You can go inside your body now, to that area of your thyroid. Imagine that you can see what that area looks like and feels like. (Pause.) Now imagine what that area looks like and feels like in its perfectly healthy state. If there is anything you would like to do to enhance the healing in that area, you can do that now. (Pause.)

As you direct your thoughts and your feelings, you can imagine accepting the experiences that come to you for your own growth and learning. You work on everything you can, and what you can't work on you leave in God's hands, knowing these are the best possible hands. As you do this you experience calmness and serenity. You find balance in actively working on all you can, recognizing that what you cannot do on your own you can release into higher hands.

This both frees and restores your energy. You go through the day feeling vitalized, energetic, confident, and serene; you go to bed at night and sleep deeply and restfully, waking up in the morning refreshed and revitalized. You can notice the energy flowing through your body, resting when you need rest and joyfully using the energy that comes to lead a meaningful and balanced life. You can see your life coming into harmony. You can see yourself as physically, mentally, and spiritually whole and vital.

Feel deep down inside to that centered place within you. That place that is strong and harmonious despite anything going on on the outside. A place of strength inside yourself. A place of comfort and safety. A place of light. And you remember that this place is always here. You know and remember that any time there is any difficulty in the outer life, that here inside is your center, your place to be at peace, to feel your serenity and strength. From this centered place now, you can feel grateful for the opportunities of life, grateful for your place in life, grateful for all those around you who love and support you, to whom you return love and support. As you send out the best in you, the best is returned.

A year later, just a few weeks before she and my father were to join me on one of my canoe retreats, my mother made an appointment for her annual exam. "There was some medication the doctor wanted to put me on last year," she said to me. "Do you remember what that was?" We had both forgotten about the prescription she'd been given.

She went in for her appointment, and the first thing Dr. Lynch asked was how she was doing on the thyroid medication. My mother explained that she'd never filled the prescription and that she felt fine. The doctor was puzzled and asked if there was anything she had done to improve the condition. "Well, I took some time to reflect on what was going on in my life, and my daughter worked with me using visualization and positive suggestions."

This was the same doctor who had been so supportive of me and had given me a clean bill of health. She was open-minded but legitimately concerned. "I realize that the emotions and the mind affect the body in many ways, but you know, Alice, the functioning of the thyroid isn't something that is affected by the mind. And to tell you the truth, I've never heard of anyone who has ever recovered a normal thyroid level without medication. I'm really interested, and I'd like to take another test to see where you're at. Is that all right with you?"

Of course, my mother was as anxious as the doctor to see what the results would show, so the test was taken. The thyroid level had moved from below normal to six points into the normal range.

I asked my mother to tell her story to the group when we were on the river. When she had finished I asked her if there was anything she was still doing. "You know there is. I send love to my thyroid all the time and thank it for the work it does for me." I also told the group about my own visualization of my cancer cells as frightened young children and how I had gone inside to embrace my cancer.

On the jet boat at the end of our trip, one of the women from our group came to sit by me and said, "I want to tell you something. I have chronic pain in my knees that I've had for years. It's never not there. It's from ski injuries and surgeries I've had over the years. When I heard you tell your story about loving your cancer and Alice sending love to her thyroid, I was very skeptical. But as I looked up at the stars that night, I decided to love my knees as an experiment. All these years I've been mad at them and at the pain, and I didn't appreciate them for how they've gotten me around. I wanted to let you know that for three days now I've been pain-free."

HEALING LAUGHTER

I came home after a long workday looking forward to a hot bath, but the flame in the old water heater on my back porch was out. I was especially tired and anxious to take a bath, so I went out to relight the pilot. I turned the gas on, but the phone rang before I could get it relit. It was getting dark when I returned and, without thinking, I struck a match so I could see the dial more clearly. I watched in what seemed like slow motion as the inside of the heater exploded and the flames shot out toward the match in my right hand, engulfing it in a fireball before putting it out.

Feeling calm and probably in shock, I went into the kitchen to examine my hand. Three fingers had turned white and felt hard, like cardboard. There was no sensation at all. I turned on the faucet to run cool water over my hand while I closed my eyes and began to visualize water running through and cooling the inside of my hand and fingers.

After several minutes I placed my hand into a large glass of cool water and went to the bathroom to check out my face in the mirror. The hair on part of my eyebrows and eyelashes and one cheek had been singed off, along with some hair on that side of my head, but otherwise my face was undamaged. It felt good to be quiet so I sat down, keeping my hand in the water and continuing to visualize coolness flowing through the inside.

Some time later my friend Randal called. I told him what had happened, and he asked if he could come over and keep me company for a while. My hand was starting to hurt so I accepted his offer, looking forward to the distraction.

As we sat talking, he noticed my face flinching from the pain and spontaneously told me a silly joke. It struck me in a belly laughing way. Then I suddenly looked at him in surprise. The pain in my hand had stopped. He started to tell me another joke, but I said, "Wait! Don't tell me another one until the pain starts again!" Every few minutes my face would begin to tense and he would tell me another joke; each time, the laughter would temporarily erase the pain. When he ran out of jokes he asked me if I'd ever heard about the silly-face contest and made an outrageous face. I went into gales of laughter that sent my pain away for a long time.

As we sat there laughing, I told Randal I was having a wonderful time and, not only that, I was glad for the accident because I'd learned something very important firsthand: that laughter is a great anesthetic. I went directly to bed after a hearty laugh and fell asleep as quickly as possible. I was barely aware of the pain starting to surface as I drifted off. When I woke up in the morning, I was surprised to find that my fingers were pink and the hardness was gone. There was a slight stiffness at first but no blisters, and the only effect from the burn was some slight cracking of my skin a few days later from dryness.

A HEALING DREAM

When Karen came to see me, she was in her early forties and working through issues of severe abuse in her childhood. She had been the youngest of several siblings and was often targeted or blamed by her older brother and sisters as the one who had "done it" if they were about to get into trouble. One sister in particular had been especially cruel to her. As an adult now, she wanted to put her past behind her and stop reacting emotionally and physically to the effects of her early abuse. Intellectually she knew that all of her siblings had suffered, as she had, and had ample cause for their own unhealthy patterns.

As soon as she was able, Karen had left home. The strength and courage she had developed in self-defense enabled her to escape her abusive situation and put herself through school, move far away from her family, and establish a successful career. Most of her siblings, including the sister who had been most cruel to her, had stayed close to home and had not broken free of the dysfunctional nature of their upbringing.

Now, an upcoming family reunion brought up many of Karen's old insecurities and fears, as well as feelings of resentment and anger toward that sister. Externally her skin had broken out into an angry red rash that she felt was directly related to her emotional state.

Karen stated her desire to stay centered in the life and awareness she had created for herself and not get pulled into old family patterns and emotions when she went back home. As she spoke, she spontaneously began to tell me about a dream she had had the night before. In it she had met her sister at a train station. They were about to take a trip together. The sister was well prepared with a lot of luggage, but as Karen looked around she realized that not only was her own suitcase gone, but her ticket was missing, too. She couldn't figure out what the dream represented, but it felt important.

Many times I've noted that our subconscious minds are so in tune with our intentions to heal the wounds of our history that the simple act of making an appointment for counseling stimulates the subconscious to begin working. The result of this inner process might come out in the form of a sudden insight before or during the session, or in certain memories that begin to surface, or in a dream such as Karen's.

The important thing, I knew, was not to attempt to interpret the dream for Karen, but to help her find the meaning for herself. Dreams often have very personal symbolic meaning, though they can also be universal. At times they can even be humorous. As I asked Karen about the lost luggage in her dream she suddenly burst out laughing. "My baggage!" she exclaimed. "I've lost my baggage! Wow, I really don't have to carry that around anymore!" Her rash began to fade and was gone in a few days.

HEALING ANGELS

"I feel so embarrassed. All the women in my classes look up to me—I'm the one who does everything right!" My mother was speaking about a tumor, possibly cancerous, that had been discovered in her colon. I reminded her of how embarrassed I had felt when I was leading retreats on how to live well and found myself with advanced cancer. "It was humiliating!"

We laughed at the absurdity of our egos—but she still had this difficult situation to face. She was now seventy-four years old, active, vital, a role model to people younger and older, and she didn't want to think that she might have to give up the quality of life she was used to.

It was my mother's intuition that had motivated her to have the test done that showed blood in her stool; a subsequent exam had revealed a suspicious-looking tumor that would need to be surgically removed. Surgery was scheduled for two weeks later. She was scared and anxious to get it over with.

My parents came prior to the surgery to enjoy a retreat at my home in the mountains. It was winter and dreary, but somehow the sun came out and poured through the cathedral-style windows in my living room that look out into the pines. I had been drawn here myself because of the inspiring and healing environment.

On Sunday morning I was doing dishes in the kitchen, not realizing that a glass had broken under the suds. When I thrust my right hand in the water, my index finger was cut open. Blood poured out. I stuck my finger under the running faucet, closing my eyes and thinking, "This bleeding has to stop."

I was aware of this thought in the background, but I wasn't focusing on it. I grabbed a cloth to wrap around my finger and went to find my mother. I told her I had been cut and that the cut was deep, and I asked her to get a bandage. When she brought it I unwrapped my hand, and to our surprise the open wound was bloodless.

We sat down to the meditation we had planned to do together and visualized being filled with a healing presence. I could feel a lot of energy and sensation in the finger I had cut. After our quiet time I took off the bandage to give it some air. The skin had already come together; it almost looked as though there were little stitches.

"I didn't know it consciously, Mom," I laughed, "but I must have cut my finger for you—for your subconscious mind to see an image of how your own body can come through surgery with very little bleeding and heal this easily and naturally."

Before surgery we had a session together in which I guided my mother in a gestalt dialogue between herself and the part of her colon that was going to be removed. She told her colon that she was sorry and that she appreciated so much all the work it had done throughout her life. When I asked her to be that part of her colon and respond, her voice became very clear and confident. "There is a time for everything," it told her, "and it's time now for me to go. It's something that just needs to be done, and I'm ready."

When the conversation was complete, I asked her if she wanted to say goodbye to her colon, and the tears rolled down her cheeks as she did. After the session she said it had felt so right to be able to say goodbye and experience her grief over the loss of that part of her body. She felt she was able now to let go.

The night before surgery I stayed at my parents' home. When they were ready for bed, I led my mother into a progressive relaxation full of positive suggestions for how her body would respond to the surgery and how quickly she could heal. She and my father, who was lying beside her, were fast asleep when I finished and turned out the lights.

"You'll do fine," we reassured her again in the morning. "Just imagine that you're surrounded by angels!" When we checked her into the hospital, a man entered the room and said, "Hi, my name is Angel Ramirez, and I'm your admitting nurse." "See," we joked, "here's one of your angels already." Then Mom stood up to get weighed, and we saw that the words "Angelica Textiles" crisscrossed over the sheets. "Look at that! Angels are everywhere!"

We went with her to the preparation room to meet the anesthesiologist. I could see the apprehension begin to cloud her face. "We need one more angel," I thought silently, as I looked around hoping to find another symbol. And there it was, right in front of me. "Read what it says on that paper dispenser on the wall," I whispered in her ear. In big letters was the word "Guardian." "You see, Mom. Even when you can't see things with your physical eyes, the universe sends symbols to remind you of how well-protected and loved you are."

In less than an hour after the surgery had started, the doctor came to find us. We could tell by his beaming face that everything had gone well. "The operation was virtually bloodless!" he exclaimed. "If we had drawn a vial of blood from her arm, we would have gotten more blood than we did during her surgery." He went on to tell us that all of her vital signs had responded perfectly.

The tumor was cancerous, as he had expected. The best outcome would be that he'd gotten it all out and that it hadn't penetrated the wall of the colon. A week later the best outcome was confirmed.

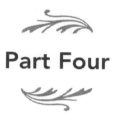

Part Four

Twelve Steps in the Healing Process

20

The Beginning of Self-Transformation

No action is more fascinating than the action of self-transformation. Nothing on earth can compare with its drama or value.

VERNON HOWARD

Looking back I can see that the greatest challenges I've encountered in life have provided the impetus that enabled me to discover my strength and to learn to trust my inner voice. They have also given me the opportunity to move my spiritual beliefs from a position of theory into a place of knowing. When I was first faced with cancer, I fell into some fear-based beliefs: that this condition symbolized some kind of failure, that healing meant getting physically well, and that I had to find out what was wrong with or bad about me if I wanted to heal.

What I had known but forgotten is that there are no failures, only lessons; that true death is living without an awareness of our spiritual nature and the beauty all around us; and that life is a school that enables us to move forward in our evolution, one grade at a time, toward God-awareness and the awakening of our own higher nature.

What I have learned is that healing isn't about living or dying; it isn't even about illness. Healing is about reconnecting to our whole-ness, and living from a foundation of love. It is about facing our deepest fears and delving deep enough to find the unique gifts that were given to us to unfold in this life.

The twelve steps that I identified on my journey through illness started out as a road map on how to die well. Since letting go of the body is something we all do at the end of life, I thought it would be useful to have some guidelines along the way. Following them taught me that dying well really amounts to living well. Right now—this present moment—is all that we ever have. It's never too late, up to our last breath, to have that one transformative understanding—that we are all spirit, all connected, all embraced in a universal unconditional love.

Looking at the soul from a perspective of ongoing growth, we come into life with a life plan. We begin with an intention to grow and heal in certain areas, both personally and collectively, but our vision is dimmed by the veils between this denser plane of physical reality and the finer plane of spiritual reality. Catastrophic events have the potential to push us beyond the habits and patterns of our dimmed awareness so that we can begin to pierce some of the veils and get on with what we're here to do—grow into conscious, aware, compassionate, and spiritual beings.

Profound healing is not a cessation of physical symptoms, but an expanded awareness of our spiritual nature. It is a process of restoring integrity to all the areas of our lives and balancing our life energy so that we're not running on a deficit. We can call on this process whenever we're confronted with a challenge, whether the challenge is in the realm of mental, emotional, or physical dis-ease, relationships, finances, or anything else. Any difficulty can serve as a wake-up call that, if we choose to heed it, directs us to an incredible supply of inner resources and strength that we might otherwise never have found.

As I confronted my own mortality, there were certain steps that I began to identify in the process of healing. There are many paths up the mountain, and we each need to discover our own; in keeping with that truth, the steps offer guidelines that can be modified in any way. They are tools to help stretch the boundaries of our consciousness and pierce the veils that limit our vision, enabling us to embrace the sacred journey of life for however long that may be, and also to prepare for the transition called death, the final adventure in this physical body. This preparation is not limited to those who have the privilege of knowing that death is imminently near. It is for all of us who realize that life is lived most fully when our loose ends are tied up, when we can be consciously whole in the present moment.

21

Step One: Take Charge

It isn't enough to pray for a miracle.
We have to take responsibility for making good choices—
life- and health-enhancing choices—and acting on them.
Once we've done all we can for ourselves, then we
can leave the results in higher hands.

CHERYL CANFIELD

My wake-up call came in the form of cancer, bringing me face-to-face with a health emergency. I found myself in the midst of a confusing, urgent swirl of diagnoses and treatment plans. Appointments were being made for me, and information was coming at me so fast I couldn't take it in. I kept hearing, "Hurry, don't wait, there is no time."

Even in the midst of the storm I knew that time was exactly what I needed. In those first weeks the only thing that seemed clear to me was that inner voice saying, "Slow down. Breathe. Your body will hold its own until you are calm enough to figure out the best path to take." I couldn't have articulated it then, but I can now assert with clarity that it isn't possible to make good, conscious decisions in the midst of confusion and shock. And so I took the first step almost blindly, following a guideline that came from inside myself: I didn't rush; even better, I slowed down. I listened to my inner voice and took charge.

It wasn't easy to step out of the pattern—or the comfort—of having someone else make the hard decisions. I had grown up in an era of passive health care, when doctors held absolute authority over treatments that we didn't understand and didn't choose. But now I realized that I was the one who had to live or die with the consequences of the treatment choices. No one else. I appreciated the expertise and experience of the team of doctors around me, but ultimately I needed to balance the options and make the decisions for myself. This meant doing much of my own research, investigating the suggestions of my medical team, and listening to my own inner responses.

Taking charge of my treatment options put me in an empowering position, but it also meant getting fully behind my decisions and my beliefs. It was something that I couldn't have done without being deeply in touch with my intuition and sense of inner guidance. I was keenly aware that each of us—I myself and every individual on my medical team—was seeing through the filter of personal history, training, and belief systems. My surgeon, for example, believed that the advanced surgical procedure he suggested represented my only chance for recovery. I had no doubt about his excellent skills and training, but my gut feeling—my intuition—told me that if I underwent the surgery I'd die on the operating table. I paid attention to this.

Doing research helped me to understand that there are many treatment options and that the experts in any given field see the benefits in terms of their particular training. Every treatment modality has some measure of success and failure (looking strictly at clearing physical symptoms). Our beliefs, because of the mind-body connection, have an impact on the way we respond to any treatment. It is also true that sometimes illness serves as a special time for us to prepare for that final journey—in which case no modality, however effective statistically, will provide a cure.

Since we can never know with certainty what a particular outcome will be, we can best use our time by choosing to live consciously and lovingly, responding to our inner sense of what is right for ourselves and our loved ones. We stay far more empowered when we take charge and make decisions that we feel good about. We can research whatever avenues we are drawn to—whether holistic, alternative, or conventional—and then choose the path or combination of modalities that supports our belief system and intuition.

Second or even third opinions can be valuable, especially when a particular suggested course raises extreme fears or doubts. To get a realistic appraisal of available treatments, we can do our own research, exploring various schools of thought. Once we've gathered information, we can make more confident treatment choices based on knowledge rather than fear.

Once a treatment plan is chosen, we can maximize its effectiveness by getting our minds and emotions into alignment with that plan. I worked with a woman named Julia who had resisted radiation for her cancer. The tumor had continued to grow until she felt she had no choice but to undergo the treatment. Yet she still thought of radiation as negatively impacting her already fragile health. She knew that this attitude would make it difficult for her body to heal, and she wanted to be more receptive. We talked about the importance of perspective and the fact that we sometimes view things rigidly as all good or all bad. But circumstances can change, and so can our perspective; the thing that seems bad from one angle can seem good from another.

I told Julia about another woman who, during her chemotherapy treatments, imagined that the chemo entered her body as light. She visualized it going through her system uncovering and clearing away all the debris. This positive image had helped her body to be receptive to the treatment; it had also successfully lessened the unpleasant side effects.

I asked Julia if she could create a positive image of the radiation treatment that would inspire her to receive it as a healing force. The tenseness in her face dissolved as she began to reframe her perspective and visualize the process in a positive way.

After her first treatment she admitted to having been scared at first, but then she said she felt a kind of peacefulness and acceptance flow through her body. "I know it sounds crazy," she told me, "but I actually found the experience interesting." With this new perspective she consciously experienced the radiation as a feeling of peacefulness that was soothing, and she responded very well. A series of treatments amazingly shrank her tumor from twelve inches in length to three, and in subsequent chemotherapy she kept all of her hair. Even though she lost weight and showed other physical signs of her ordeal, she developed an incredible emotional strength and joyfulness.

22

Step Two: Develop an Empowered Attitude

Everything can be taken from a man but one thing; the last of human freedoms—to choose one's attitude in any given set of circumstances, to choose one's own way.

VICTOR FRANKL

A certain attitude emerged in New Age thought that we create our own illness. Of course we are subject to the consequences of poor choices. If we smoke, for example, we're gambling with the possibility of lung cancer. We also know that strong emotions can create chemical reactions in the body that can have certain physical effects. Laughter and love, on the positive side, are said to release endorphins and chemicals that boost the immune system and create a sense of well-being. Ongoing resentment, rage, and grief, on the other hand, deplete the immune system and can lead to illness or debility in some area.

But when we find ourselves confronted with a life-threatening illness, it is disempowering and guilt producing to be charged with having created it. This attitude has devastated many individuals already struggling with a major challenge. A catastrophic illness or other life challenge can become a great catalyst that moves us forward. As I once heard Caroline Myss put it, illness can be the answer to a prayer. We don't set out to create cancer, but when it happens we can receive it (if we choose to do the inner work) as an opportunity to learn and grow.

An empowered attitude always results when we're in sync with inner guidance; we experience a sense of rightness. As I worked on my own healing, I heeded that sense in even the smallest decisions. If something didn't feel right, I didn't do it, and I kept my rational mind out of it.

The rational mind is that part that jumps in after an intuition and takes us in circles, leading us away from the clarity the intuition brought. The more we acknowledge and pay attention to that initial intuitive feeling, even if logic would question its validity, the stronger our intuition becomes.

Whenever we face any difficulty or challenge, we have an opportunity to learn, to grow, or to be of service in some way. A particular illness or condition or experience of lack may be a response to our own request for healing in some area of our life. And it's not uncommon for adverse situations to open a whole new pathway in life or to add a new dimension in our relationship to God, to ourselves, or to others. It takes patience and trust. We don't ordinarily see the lessons we're working on when we're in the middle of them. Insight usually comes in retrospect and grows and develops through time.

Developing an empowered attitude requires a conscious effort to change any habits that make us feel weak, overwhelmed, or powerless. Three common areas that we can all work on toward greater emporwerment are words, feelings, and body language.

We use words in both our speech and our thoughts. Many of us have picked up unhealthy expressions that actually bring us down or block us from the things we are capable of achieving. The word *can't* is a good example. If we think we can't do something, we probably won't do it. But if we think we can, we may surprise even ourselves in finding that we really can.

When my former husband and I were building our own house, I assumed we would need to bring in an electrician to do the wiring. I brought up the question of whom we might hire, and my father, who was helping that day, said, "Just buy a book and do it yourself." He said it so matter-of-factly that I just assumed I would be able to do it—and so I did. I bought a book, studied the diagrams and codes, designed each circuit on paper, and went to work. When the wiring was completed, it was astounding to me that the lights actually went on at the flick of a switch. I felt very empowered. If I'd thought I couldn't do it, I never would have tried.

When you find yourself using the word *can't*, try substituting the word *won't* and notice how the energy shifts; now, you're taking responsibility in the situation. "I can't carry that heavy basket!" becomes a lot more empowering when you change it to "I won't carry that heavy basket." Now you're making a conscious choice.

You can try the same thing with *should*, another disempowering word. *Should* is laden with guilt. "I should clean the house," or "I really should go on a diet." Be empowered. "The house needs cleaning, but I want to go to that event. I'll clean it tomorrow," or "I'd love to lose some weight, but I'm not ready to commit. After the holidays I'll get serious." These are examples of empowered choices—but it's important to act on the choices you make. If you decide to put something off until another time, follow through when the time arrives. You'll be surprised at how confident and powerful you become.

The second area that strongly affects our sense of empowerment is the realm of feelings. I remember that sadness and fear used to attack me in the middle of the night. I'd wake up and those awful feelings would wash over me or grab me in the stomach. I dreaded it. This signaled the beginning, sometimes, of hours of miserable insomnia as my emotions went on to engage my mind in one drab mental scenario after another. It was very disempowering.

Over time I started to realize that if I allowed myself to be quiet and simply feel the feeling, its source would usually reveal itself. And when I thought about it, feelings of both sadness and fear usually had to do with something that had already happened or that might never happen. The few fears that were realized over the course of my illness released their hold on me as I dealt with them in the moment. In one way or another, I was able to resolve whatever it was that triggered the feelings, and the dread disappeared.

My challenge became how to get through the dark nights without churning up all that emotional discomfort. I found many creative solutions. The little dog I'd had was now gone and the feral cat who had been living on my roof moved inside and became a great comforter in the night. It would have been hard not to resonate to the soothing sound of Socrates purring; all it required to get his motor humming were a few strokes along his soft furry body. Inspirational guided meditation tapes provided another way to set my mind in a more positive direction until morning's light, when I always felt more grounded and able to deal with things.

TOP DOG

Feels Superior • Makes Judgments
Has to Be Right • Doesn't Admit to Mistakes
Holds Grudges • Competes for Power & Control
Manipulates Others • Uses Intimidation & Humiliation
Likes to be Center Stage • Often Feels Isolated from Others

EGO IDENTIFICATION

VICTIM CONSCIOUSNESS

Feels Unimportant • Lacks a Sense of Self-Worth and Value
Is Easily Manipulated or Controlled • Feels Powerless
Lacks Confidence • Looks to Others for Direction
Is Overly Sensitive or Thin-Skinned
Often Feels Anxious or Depressed

UNDERDOG

Disempowering Ego Attitudes

Another important tool was my journal. In the night I would make lists of everything I could think of that made me feel good and uplifted, everything that I was grateful for in my life. Then during the day, when my mind was clearer and more centered, I used my journal to help process the feelings that came up at night. As I gained confidence, through many experiences, that I could change the way I felt at night by changing my focus, it became easier to release my fears.

The third area of empowerment is body language. The way we hold and move our bodies can make a dramatic difference in how we approach things. When I'm feeling down or disempowered, I stretch my arms overhead, reaching way up with my fingertips. Then I open my palms upward and imagine receiving energy and grace from that

Loving

Forgives and Moves On

Has a Sense of Personal Power

Inner-Directed • Confident • Optimistic

Sees Problems as Opportunities to Learn and Grow

Faces Life Squarely • Makes Conscious Choices

SPIRITUAL IDENTIFICATION

Sees Self as Part of the Whole • Works for the Good of All

Balances Personal Needs with the Needs of Others

Admits Mistakes and Learns from Them

Is Compassionate Toward All Life

Has a Sense of Purpose

Feels Worthy

Empowering Spiritual Attitudes

endless universal source. Simple actions like this can make a perceptible difference.

If you're slumping as you sit or stand, try pulling your shoulders back. Notice the difference. And breathe. When we're tense we're usually holding our breath or breathing shallowly. Focused physical movement and deep, slow breathing can literally change our feelings. Doing yoga postures with a focus on keeping the spine straight, standing or sitting tall, and opening the chest while breathing—all can make a profound difference. So can getting out into nature and walking with shoulders back and head high.

An empowered attitude is an unshakable knowing that you are centered and strong: whatever the circumstances, you can and will find a way to keep or regain that sense of centeredness and strength within yourself.

23

Step Three: Create a Healing Environment

*Discover the joy in the now, some of the peace in the here,
some of the love in me and thee which go to make up
the kingdom of heaven on earth.*

ANNE MORROW LINDBERGH

BUILDING THE INNER FOUNDATION

A healing environment is the foundation from which we can live our lives more fully present and alive, and the place to start constructing that environment is within. The principle in the expression, "as above, so below," can find another expression in "as within, so without." When our minds are cluttered, our external environment tends to become cluttered.

A woman once told me that her elderly mother, who suffered from dementia, had good days and bad days. A good day meant that her mind was fairly clear, and a bad day meant that she was very disoriented. The woman noted a consistent pattern: on the days when her mother's mind was clear, her purse was well organized. When she was disoriented, her purse was full of clutter.

Everything in our experience is influenced by the state of our mind, and the state of our mind is something that we have some control over.

The mind is the first place where change begins. To create order out of chaos when our thinking becomes depressed or disjointed or chaotic, we can begin by building an inner sanctuary, a place we can retreat to at any time to reconnect with our centeredness and grounding.

Whether our practice is meditation or prayer or quiet time alone, any practice is most effectively integrated into our lives by putting aside a certain time for it each day. Returning to the same place at the same time creates an automatic cue for relaxation and promotes a deepening of the experience. If you think you have no time or place to relax undisturbed, switch from showers to baths and let bath time be your quiet time. If you can't put aside thirty minutes or an hour each day for yourself, you've lost balance and need to rework your priorities to include essential quiet time alone.

Relaxing the body is the best way to enter into a practice when it is not already an established habit. Turn off the phone or do whatever you need to do to avoid distractions, and find a comfortable place to sit with your head supported and your legs and arms uncrossed to allow energy to flow freely. Give yourself anywhere from ten to thirty minutes in the beginning, setting your internal alarm or choosing some other signal to let you know when the time is up.

The breath is the first bridge to relaxation. Taking several deep, slow breaths, holding them briefly and then blowing out, automatically signals the body to slow down. The next step is simply to allow the breath to become slow and comfortable and easy. At first the mind may want to keep jumping around; it can help to imagine thoughts coming in and flowing out without paying them much attention. The idea is not to fight against thinking, but just to notice the thoughts and keep bringing your awareness back to the breath.

Once some level of relaxation is reached, we can use the mind to begin to create a wonderful inner sanctuary. This becomes the foundation of our inner healing environment. An inner sanctuary is as unique as each individual, so what follows are suggestions to get the creative juices flowing.

To be most effective, the imagination can involve as many senses as possible. If the scene being created is a beautiful garden in nature, brilliant colors and scents can be brought in, a gentle breeze ruffling leaves or the chirping of birds can be imagined. Texture can be incorporated by imagining the feel of a fallen leaf or a smooth, cool rock or the sifting of warm grains of sand through our fingers. We can imagine tasting the rainwater trapped on a velvety leaf or opening our mouths to catch a spray from a nearby waterfall. There is no limit to our creative imaginations. We can bring in anything that lifts us up and opens our hearts. With consistent repetition this imaginative inner environment becomes an empowering and healing place that can be returned to again and again. And when we become very comfortable we can slip into quiet, receptive stillness.

There is no right way to be quiet. Setting the time aside each day and keeping it is success enough. Whatever happens is right. Once the state of inner quiet becomes established, it can be recalled at any time or place. Since inspirations and insights come during quiet moments, I keep writing pads handy around my "quiet places" and sometimes take a pad and pen with me on my walking meditations in nature. Just as dreams sometimes fade when we wake up, new ideas can fade from our conscious minds if we don't make note of them. And if we don't move our inspirations into action, they become unrealized potential. Inspiration is part of our inner guidance system, directing us toward the higher path of our soul's journey. We reach our goals when we act on the guidance that comes.

AS WITHIN, SO WITHOUT

A healing environment is also something we can create externally in any space that we have control over—our work and home environments—consciously making them into places that inspire us, lift our spirits, and connect us with our hearts. Heart energy is a powerful source of healing. Pay attention to the things that uplift you—colors, sounds, textures, photos, mementos, and so on. Keep yourself surrounded by the things you love.

I remember a story about a woman who invited a Feng Shui consultant into her home. She had been divorced for several years and now wanted to be in another relationship, but things weren't working out for her in that way. When the consultant walked into the bedroom, she asked the woman how she felt about the big, dark wooden furniture that occupied the space. "Every time I walk in here I think of my ex-husband," she said. "This bedroom set was something I got in the divorce settlement. When I look at it I think at least I got something good out of a lousy marriage." The consultant advised her to get rid of it and replace it with furniture that reflected more of herself. The woman did so. Not surprisingly, when she stopped being reminded every day of the "lousy marriage" she'd had, she found a good relationship in no time.

Creating a physical environment that uplifts and supports us isn't just about image, or what a space looks like; it's about energy, or how a space feels to us. Objects in our environment may be beautiful, but if they keep us tied to feelings that weight us down or hold us back, they can actually be draining our energy and diminishing the quality of our lives.

Most of us are more "clairsentient"—aware of the energy of people and things around us—than we realize. Take a look around the rooms you spend a lot of time in and begin testing out your intuitive senses. How do you feel when you come into a particular room? Notice what gets your attention, and then notice whether the feeling it evokes is uplifting or heavy, or if it makes you happy or sad. Look at different objects and continue to evaluate them in this way. When you tune into your feelings, you might be surprised. It may be time to get rid of those "status" things you never liked, or the representations of the past that you're still holding on to. Bring in more living energy, like plants or beautiful art or colors or whatever fills you with vitality and joy.

Besides surrounding ourselves with positive, uplifting things, simplifying our external environment can also be good therapy. Cleaning out closets, drawers, attics, or any space in our domain helps us to feel clear and light. Passing on the things we're not using to someone who needs them gives us an opportunity to do a good deed at the same time. As we let go of outer clutter, we may find that it gets easier to let go of inner clutter.

24

Step Four: Practice Forgiveness

Here is a mental treatment guaranteed to cure every ill that flesh
is heir to: sit for half an hour every night and mentally forgive
everyone against whom you have any ill will or antipathy.

CHARLES FILLMORE

PATH TO PERSONAL FREEDOM

Forgiveness is often one of the hardest things to practice, but it is a powerful means of personal transformation. Forgiving and letting go doesn't mean condoning the hurtful or violent actions of others. It means that we no longer allow ourselves to be victims of those actions by holding them to us. Although it can be a holy or altruistic act, forgiveness is more often an act of self-empowerment, as it frees us from the bonds that tie us so we can move on.

When we forgive we are saying, in essence, that we are no longer willing to carry around pain in response to someone else's actions. This drains our energy, as do feelings of guilt or blame toward ourselves. We can take that same energy and put it to use in a positive direction. As we let go of bitterness and guilt, the heart energy that we've been blocking begins to flow more freely, allowing us to give and receive the love we desire and need.

In metaphysics the heart chakra sits in the middle of the lower and the higher chakras, like a gateway between the two. The lower chakras have to do with the physical world, where it's possible to be treated and cured from a medical standpoint. But to heal on every level and to fully activate the higher chakras, such as compassion and insight and wisdom, it is necessary to open the heart; that requires the experience of forgiveness.

Forgiveness is a core life lesson. It means cutting the cord of resentment we have attached to another person and trusting God or Spirit to bring that person the experiences he or she needs to heal. When we harbor thoughts of vengeance or resentment, we aren't hurting anyone but ourselves. And if we want to be free to heal, we have to learn how to cut those cords.

When I was going through the forgiveness phase in my healing process, I used many techniques, including writing dialogues in my journal, as I described in chapter five—conversations between myself and anyone I could think of toward whom I had even the slightest resentment. It is possible to make an instant connection with the highest spiritual energy—compassion—and experience an immediate cessation of blame and guilt and resentment. Though this energy is always available to us there are times when we're not ready for it. At those times, I accepted the sincerity of my desire to forgive and be free, and imagined lifting the burden up to God to hold for me. I didn't have to carry guilt over my lack of compassion because it was in higher hands until I was ready to forgive. I call it "practicing forgiveness" because sometimes the anger or the resentment or the bitterness we feel toward a particular situation or person may come back, and we have to keep lifting it back up until we are able to let it go completely.

The practice of forgiveness is something that can be cultivated into a lifelong response to whatever difficult feelings and situations come up. The lessons we learn from each encounter help us in the struggle to keep our hearts open. It isn't only personal situations that affect us, but the collective experiences of humanity. Each one of us is responsible, through our actions or lack of action, in helping to determine the direction of the greater whole.

One of the most powerful tools I've found to keep my heart open to compassion and forgiveness is to direct my thoughts outward with a positive intention. Even when I'm not able to do anything else, I can hold individuals or situations (especially those I have difficulty with) in a place of compassion. I do this in my quiet time each day, and the practice helps me to keep the energy that I project into the world positive. I use the following visualization:

Imagine a golden light radiating down from above; a light of healing and compassion and wisdom. I breathe the light in with my breath. The golden light circulates throughout my body, focussing especially on any area that needs attention or healing. As my body fills with light it overflows through my heart chakra. I reach out with this heart energy and touch the hearts of my loved ones and friends—and especially anyone or anything that I'm feeling critical of. As the light expands I imagine reaching out as a group and touching the hearts of all those in the world who feel hopelessness or despair or whose hearts are hardened or cold. We further expand the light, reaching out into the hearts of all individuals and groups in the world whose power and influence impacts us all. Finally I visualize lifting the earth up into God's hands with my prayer that humanity, individually and collectively, come into harmony with our highest good and the good of the whole.

With our hearts clear and our thoughts compassionate, we can act as a powerful force in the world. We are all needed in the important work of forgiveness and healing.

Forging the Future

Lack of forgiveness on a national level is as devastating as it is on an individual level. The lessons are everywhere to be seen. Bitter battles are being fought around the world as one nation lashes out against another and the other lashes back. The violence—along with the attending physical and emotional devastation—is perpetuated through endless decades of holding on to anger and rage. Walls are built up and habits of thinking become so deeply entrenched that forgiveness becomes an unthinkable concept.

And yet forgiveness is the only path that will clear away the revenge and rage that feed the escalating violence. Just as in personal or domestic violence, perpetrators on either side need to be stopped and the innocent need to be protected—by laws, by the non-violent actions of freedom-loving people of the world, and by nations coming together in solidarity and cooperation.

In every situation that confronts us, individually or collectively, we have a choice as to whether we will respond from our lower natures—from a position of fear or anger that posits a top dog against an underdog—or from our higher natures, from an empowered position of compassion and integrity. When we respond from the side of fear, we often choose short-term solutions that compromise higher principles in order to achieve a goal; such is the case when we sanction the killing of fellow human beings for political means. As we sacrifice the values we hold dear, we mimic that which we detest. When our hearts are thus hardened, we suffer the debilitating consequences: principles get compromised, truth becomes distorted, and apathy becomes pervasive. When we respond from the side of compassion, we tend to choose long-term solutions that protect our principles, ensuring that our actions demonstrate our integrity and allow us to mature toward our highest potentials. The philosophy of violence, that the end justifies the means, is contributing to the mental and physical deterioration of individuals and countries. It is making us sick. The philosophy of compassion, that only a just means leads to a just end, can make us well.

As we look to heal our lives, we need to reclaim the integrity of our words and actions. Every time we act from our highest values, we are not only healing ourselves, we are also helping to heal the world. We need to speak and act in ways that heal, not ways that hurt, lest we ourselves become the victims. As we forgive ourselves and others, we unlock the door that leads to true freedom.

25

Step Five:
Explore Attitudes and Beliefs

All belief that does not make us more happy, more free,
more loving, more active, more calm, is, I fear,
a mistaken and superstitious belief.

JOHN K. LAVATER

Beliefs and attitudes can become so embedded in our subconscious minds that it's easy to lose track of them. We can even hold conflicting beliefs without being aware of it. Asking questions, I discovered, helped me to identify certain underlying beliefs that weakened rather than strengthened me. When we connect with that quiet inner place, we find that we have access inside to the answers we need; often, the right questions can lead us there.

I turned to meditation and then to my journal to start formulating questions. At first they were general: "Who am I?" and "What am I doing here?" Philosophical questions such as these give us a broader perspective and can help us begin to identify the beliefs that govern our attitudes and reactions to the circumstances around us.

At other times I found that certain questions, such as, "Why is this happening to me?" brought me into a state of helplessness. When we're in the middle of an emotional and difficult situation, we rarely have the perspective to know why. Not only is it a frustrating and unanswerable question, but it also reveals a victim attitude.

On the other hand, when questions call for action on our part, they become empowering and get us moving. The more we confront our underlying disempowering beliefs and attitudes, the more opportunity we have to turn them around. Once I realized that, I changed the question to, "If me, why?" I had cancer. That was a fact. What was I going to do with it? The more specific my questions became, the clearer the answers that followed.

In my counseling work with individuals, people often begin by telling me that they don't know what to do in a particular situation. They might be making a decision about a treatment or a relationship; it doesn't matter. Usually within a few minutes of my asking questions, they're telling me the answer to what they previously were sure they didn't know. When I point this out, we laugh.

One of the things that sometimes throws us off is that we unconsciously judge our decisions based on how others might feel about them or how they might perceive us. As an example, a woman had recently had a mastectomy. Two doctors were recommending radiation as a follow-up procedure, but she wasn't sure it was the right decision. As I questioned her, it came out that she strongly felt the radiation treatment was right for her. Her doubt came from the fact that her husband's opinion differed from hers. She wanted the assurance that she felt the radiation would give her, but she was concerned that her husband's opinion might be better than her own. In the end she decided to follow her intuition, which was to go ahead with the treatment.

Our lives become very complicated when we look to other people's beliefs to tell us what we need to do, or when we hold our own beliefs as best for someone else. When we straighten out the boundaries, it becomes much easier to get to that place of knowing within. We all have inner guidance; but no matter how close our relationship to another might be, our guidance applies only to ourselves. Of course, parents use their own guidance where minor children are concerned. It takes maturity to discern when a child's individual perspective is valid for making sound decisions.

The words we use to communicate are symbols of our internal beliefs. As I found myself saying and writing things that felt disempowering, I discovered attitudes within myself that didn't support healing. As I consciously reframed these negative beliefs and changed certain images and words, negative habit patterns started to dissolve.

Most of us pick up a mixture of positive and negative impressions about ourselves and the world. How common it is to hear someone say, for example, "Whenever things get too good, I know something bad is going to happen." Expectations tend to be realized, so we might as well set them on the positive side.

I even discovered that certain supposedly positive words convey ideas that in reality contain negative suggestions. The word *remission* is an example. Whenever anyone asks if my cancer is in remission, I always say, "Heavens, no! Remission is like having something hanging over your shoulder ready to pounce on you. I don't know what's going to happen tomorrow or next year. I only know that today I'm well."

I continue to pay attention to my thoughts and to the words I use because they reflect the beliefs I choose. Whenever I realize that I'm thinking or speaking in a way that holds me back or causes me to think less of myself or someone else, I realize I have an opportunity to reframe a limiting belief into something that empowers me and the people around me. As Norman V. Peale put it, "Change your thoughts and you change your world."

We create through thought. When we take hold of that as a spiritual belief, we get in touch with our potential to be a positive influence in the world. And though a spiritual motive isn't self-serving, we can't give without receiving. When we give out positive energy, we get back positive energy in return.

Empowering or spiritual attitudes and beliefs are centered in our highest good and in the good of the whole. They enhance physical, emotional, and spiritual well-being. Disempowering or aggrandizing attitudes and beliefs are centered in the lower self, or ego, where perceptions are framed in terms of top dog versus underdog. When we allow this part of ourselves to be in charge, it's like putting a child at the head of the family. The results are detrimental to physical, emotional, and spiritual well-being. Developing spiritual awareness leads to a recognition of these two aspects of ourselves so that we can consciously put the higher discerning mind in charge, allowing us to keep our balance and perspective:

LOWER SELF		HIGHER SELF
Thinks in terms of comfort and convenience for the body	→	Thinks in terms of psychological and spiritual well-being
Sees itself as the center of the universe	→	Sees itself as one cell in the body of humanity
Is self-centered, concerned with personal gain	→	Has a selfless balance, is concerned with the good of the whole
Makes judgments, distinctions, and separations	→	Applies discernment, strives for unity and oneness
Operates under the law of aggression	→	Operates under the law of love
Has a competitive nature	→	Has a cooperative nature

Many of our attitudes come from beliefs we formulated about ourselves and the world around us when we were very young and had not yet developed reasoning minds. We observed and listened and took on various attitudes that were greatly influenced by our parents, teachers, and by society in general. Most of us picked up a mixed jumble of positive and negative beliefs based on our early subjective experiences and interpretations.

A single careless remark taken in at an early age can get into our subconscious and continue to influence our experiences throughout our lives—unless it is consciously recognized and released. For example, children can absorb a comment (sometimes misinterpreted) that they are stupid or unattractive or will never succeed, and they grow into adulthood believing this, whether consciously or not, and acting it out in their lives. Or an early traumatic experience can take hold, leaving a child feeling responsible or guilty or somehow "bad." Underlying feelings may persist even when the memories have faded.

The purpose of examining our attitudes is not to trace our difficulties back to some outside source and put blame there, but to recognize that we picked up misconceptions when we were young and that as adults we can change those misconceptions. For example, if I have lived my life with the subconscious belief that I will never succeed and can now recognize this as a false belief, a misconception that I took on at some point, then I have an opportunity to change the pattern of my experience. Bad things may have happened when we were children; but we can change the influence they have on us if we're willing to look for something positive to take from the experience. I knew a man once who had accumulated a great deal of wealth, only to lose it all during the depression. His attitude was one of acceptance. "Well, I made it once, I can do it again." In five years he rebuilt his wealth. Another man who lost his wealth at the same time fell into despair and took his own life. He lost the opportunity to learn and grow that is always available to us.

If we want to be at our strongest, it's important to find ways to move from helplessness to acceptance, with the courage to continue on. We may not be able to control the circumstances outside of us, but we can and do retain control over our attitudes and responses to outside events. It isn't possible to understand everything that happens. No explanation can dissolve the pain that a parent feels at the loss of a child, for instance. But we can accept that we have only a small view of the big picture. Even grief can move us to do something healing for ourselves and the world.

Many have found strength by allowing their grief to motivate them to comfort others suffering from loss. Foundations that serve thousands of others have been set up in honor of a departed loved one. Turning our grief into good works doesn't cancel out the pain of separation, but it can further strengthen our bonds with those who have passed on before us and ease our loneliness.

Our attitudes can and do color our perception of the world and our experiences in life.

⤜ **26** ⤛

Step Six:
Transform Negative Feelings—
Heal and Release the Past

A lake that is absolutely calm gives to you a perfect reflection.
The moment it becomes disturbed in the least, the reflection
is distorted; and if the agitation is increased, the reflection
will be completely lost. Your consciousness is the lake.

JAMES B. SCHAFER

The present is the only time we ever really have; if we don't live in the present, we don't even scratch the surface of our potential. Two common negative feelings that keep us out of the present are guilt and worry. Guilt keeps us stuck in the past, losing energy over something that already happened. Worry is a nonproductive mulling over of some negative possibility in the future that may never happen. When we find ourselves in either of those states, we can switch our focus to concern, which is something we can act on in the present to either heal the past or influence the future in a positive way.

Paying attention to how we spend our energy can provide major clues in the process of healing. Certain emotions, such as blame, guilt, anger, or fear, that we return to again and again, can literally drain our life force and leave little or nothing to fuel the immune system.

Unlike the burst of fear or adrenaline that temporarily fires us up to respond quickly in an emergency situation—a kind of energy that is easily replenished—the ongoing burdens of guilt and blame over "what was" or fear of "what may be" is draining. Holding on to negative feelings is simply an exhausting expenditure of energy that can lead to emotional and physical bankruptcy.

We cannot become self-aware unless we consciously choose to identify our habit patterns, which begin with our thoughts. Are you generally positive in your thinking? Do you think of your cup as half full or half empty? If your immediate response was on the positive, full side, does it hold up under examination?

I was once having a conversation with a friend in which I was adamant that there was only one course of action open to me in a particular situation. "You're pretty rigid in your thinking about this," he said to me. His comment momentarily stunned me, as I prided myself on being flexible and open in my thinking. It gave me pause. Later, I realized he was right. I had fallen into black-and-white thinking in this particular instance.

We cannot change our patterns unless and until we become aware of them. Establishing a habit of regular journaling can provide an excellent way to expand awareness and work on positive change. When we're feeling stuck, we may benefit from the objective guidance of a good counselor.

When we hold bitterness or anger or fear toward another, we hurt ourselves, not the object of our focus. We drain our own energy, and this affects us on all levels. Further, through our bitter focus we grow our adversary into the proportions of a giant or a monster. When we let go of damaging negative emotions and the stories that feed them, our adversaries tend to shrink. In time, they may even disappear altogether.

Unconscious or submerged issues can also drain our vitality. It takes a lot of psychic energy to keep old traumas from our conscious awareness; expenditures of this kind are equally exhausting and depleting. But if we aren't aware of these buried problems, how do we know if we have them? Although they may be difficult to get in touch with, certain clues may point to their existence. These include ongoing mild depression or a sense that we're blocking ourselves or that we sabotage ourselves from meeting certain goals. Again, journaling or counseling can begin to bring the issues that we haven't been ready to deal with to the surface.

One man who came to see me, Bill, had prostate cancer that had metastasized to his bones. He had been struggling with this condition for five years, using both conventional and alternative medicine. When I first saw him, he had decided that the time had come to focus on the spiritual side of his life. I told him that the spiritual path was not an easy path. It takes courage to know ourselves honestly and hard work to make whatever changes may be necessary.

He was eager to begin and took copious notes as we spoke. Between our next few meetings, Bill made trips to various treatment clinics where he did everything possible to get his cancer under control. His attitude was optimistic most of the time; he was learning to use meditation and relaxation, however sporadically, to pull himself out of occasional depressions. But I sensed that he wasn't really getting in touch with his emotions. He gently brushed off any difficulties in his personal relationships and seemed disconnected from his wife and young children.

After several meetings he brought up the fact that he had never dealt with or grieved the death of his parents. They had been dead now for ten years. The pain was obvious in Bill's face as he went back to the particularly painful death of his mother only months after his father was killed in an accident. His emotions spilled out in cathartic release as he told the story.

As I guided him into a dialogue between his mother and himself, it came out that he felt a tremendous amount of responsibility toward her, and guilt that he had somehow failed her. Periodically during the dialogue I would ask him to imagine switching to the objective perspective of his higher self. From there, Bill talked about various misconceptions he had developed about the demands and responsibilities he had heaped on himself.

Through the dialogue his mother also expressed disappointments about some of his choices in life. As they went on, they began to come to the understanding that as a young man he had needed to make his own choices and to do what was right for him. As the dialogue came to a conclusion, she gave Bill her blessings and acceptance.

I asked him if there was anything else he would like to say to his mother. "Mom, I can't come and be with you now. I have to stay here and take care of my family." She replied, "Yes, son, you need to be there for them just as I was there for you. I love you and I will always love you and I'm here for you whenever you need me." For the first time since her death, Bill felt free of the guilt that had been pulling him out of the present and draining his life energy.

This awareness of the life force as energy is key to the vision of profound healing. If we don't change the pattern of negative expenditures of energy, we'll continue to come up with a deficit that manifests again and again in the same symptoms or new ones. To really heal we need to open up to the transforming power of compassion and forgiveness, both toward ourselves and others. This power connects us to that universal source, through which our energy is ever replenished. Then we can transcend the temporary cessation of symptoms that is sometimes taken for healing.

In a study designed to measure immune responses, a group of people were asked to spend twenty minutes a day for one week writing about the most traumatic event in their lives. Comparing the results against a control group, researchers found that those who wrote about their trauma had much stronger immune responses. It's healthy to pull up the traumas from our past, sometimes stored unconsciously, and release them.

As we heal and release the past, we are released from the charge we have given to certain events. They lose their power over us, and we can better learn the lessons inherent in them. When we have a healthy relationship with and understanding of the past, we can visit it without getting stuck there or falling back into the position of a victim.

27

Step Seven:
Build a Support System

*If a patient is denied the opportunity to discuss what is
most troubling—fear, pain, death—he or she will feel isolated.
When what really matters to you is precisely what you
cannot discuss, then you are very lonely indeed.*

O. CARL SIMONTON

It's common to feel isolated when facing a life-threatening or debilitating condition, even when surrounded by loved ones. I had many scary thoughts, but I didn't want to express them to the people who loved me and worried about me. I needed and appreciated the support I got from my family and friends, but I also needed support from more neutral sources who could hear what I was feeling without being hurt or shocked. A supportive counselor can be invaluable, as can a support group with empowering guidelines.

No matter how much we empathize with someone facing a difficult challenge, only those who are facing or who have faced something similar can convey a sense of real and deep knowing. Many studies have shown that people in support groups cope better. For example, individuals in cancer support groups who receive identical treatments to those in control groups without support have been shown to have longer survival rates. Being with others who share the experience can provide a sense of community, along with new information and varying perspectives. The emotional support from such a group can offer people in crisis a connection to life and help them through the rough places, as well as prepare them for the possibility of death. What we all ultimately learn is that life is temporary in any case; from that, hopefully, we take in that every moment is a moment to be treasured.

Along with outer support I found that building a core of inner support helped me move into an active and strong role in my healing process. Journaling helped me to find a best friend in myself, and meditation connected me to God and my sense of higher guidance.

I learned to confide in and talk over important decisions only with family, friends, and professionals who could support me by accepting and rallying behind my choices, whether they agreed with me or not. For example, my daughter, Cindy, once told me, "Mom, I couldn't make the choices you're making, but if anyone can do it, you can." Her words touched me profoundly and gave me a sense of confidence. True support is always empowering. On the other hand we are sometimes confronted by loved ones, who, albeit with good intention, try to sabotage our efforts or dissuade us from our choices when they don't agree with them. As difficult as it may be, and especially when we're experiencing major illness or crisis in our lives, it's essential to set personal boundaries and learn to communicate in ways that keep us empowered to remain true to ourselves.

Of course this practice helps to prevent emotional and physical distress from the start. When we know we can trust ourselves to communicate truthfully and make decisions that are in sync with our inner guidance, our emotions and bodies remain clear and empowered. As we honor our need to be in charge of our own lives, we learn to honor the rights of those we're close to, so that we can experience truly supportive relationships.

Part of the difficulty in setting personal boundaries—and setting them is essential to our outer and inner support system—is that many of us were conditioned with such distorted boundaries while growing up that we have no idea what healthy boundaries look like.

The following are signs of a lack of healthy boundaries:

- Needing to camouflage our feelings or being afraid to tell the truth in our personal relationships
- Needing to control other people or allowing ourselves to be controlled by others
- Thinking in rigid or inflexible ways; seeing only black and white, or acknowledging only one way to do something—our way!
- Being swayed by the opinions or actions of others because we want to feel like part of the group or be accepted by another
- Depending on another person's perspective to represent us when we're giving an opinion
- Being unable to say no when we're asked to do something that we don't want to do or that infringes on other responsibilities
- Being motivated to do things so that people will like us

The following are signs of healthy boundaries:

- Being able to communicate our feelings without putting blame outside of ourselves or taking on guilt
- Taking responsibility for making our own choices, and supporting our family members and friends in their choices, even when they differ from ours
- Respecting the opinions of others and being willing to look at the other side with an open mind
- Having the strength to stick with the opinions or choices that we know are right for us
- Trusting the worth of our own ideas and opinions

- Knowing when to say no and having the ability to say it
- Feeling passion for the things we do because we enjoy doing them

The basis of healthy boundaries is respect—both for ourselves and for others.

28

Step Eight:
Simplify Life

*When we do a mental and spiritual inventory of all that we
have, we realize that we are very rich indeed. Grattitude gives
way to simplicity—the desire to clear out, pare down, and
realize the essentials of what we need to live truly well.*

SARAH BAN BREATHNACH

Our lives are often so cluttered and busy that we find ourselves racing
to keep up. We lose the simple basics that provide the balance we so
desperately need: walks in nature, unhurried time with our loved
ones, precious quiet time alone for meditation or reading or simply
being mindfully grateful for the many gifts around us.

What it means to simplify life is different for each individual. For
me, the process began with finding the courage to leave the chaotic
situation I was in, which included a relationship with a partner who
wasn't willing to participate in counseling. When I told my husband
before I was diagnosed with cancer that our conflicts were killing me,
I meant it metaphorically, as a description of my growing feeling of
helplessness over the deteriorating communication between us. But
the sense of being killed played out literally in my life, a vivid
reminder of the connection between the mind, body, and spirit.

213

On a very basic level, simplifying life can mean clearing out the physical environment—going through closets and anywhere things are stashed and giving away what isn't being used and probably never will be. If I've stored something for a year without missing it, or if I haven't worn a piece of clothing in that time, I figure I'm ready to let it go. It's a good rule in general. Pass on the things that clutter up your space to someone who can really use them.

Peace Pilgrim told a story about a woman whose house burned down. She and her husband had been living in the big home they had raised their family in, and after the fire they moved into a house more suitable for just the two of them. Peace started to sympathize with the woman but she stopped her, saying, "Now I'll never have to clean out those closets, and I'll never have to clean out that attic." In telling the story Peace remarked, "But wouldn't it have been better if they had learned to give and had extended their surplus toward those who needed it? Then they would have been blessed by the giving, and others would have been blessed by the getting."

Many of us become so used to the things that are tying us down that we don't realize we've lost our freedom. Work is one of those areas. How many people are working at jobs they hate in order to put food on the table?

One man who came to see me worked in real estate. As the years had gone by, he had become more and more depressed. He really wanted to start his own business, but out of guilt that he might not hold up his end financially he never allowed himself to think it through or discuss it with his wife. When he finally got the courage to talk to her about his passion, he was amazed at how receptive she was to his ideas. She assured him that they could afford to live on her income until his business was established. When I saw him two years later, he was happily pursuing his new career. He and his wife had moved to a more modest house that they both loved, and their relationship had grown closer than ever as enthusiasm for life replaced his previous depression.

Another person who came to see me was running a successful business with her husband but felt stressed and overwhelmed. The hours were long, and many of the tough responsibilities fell to her. She felt competent in her work but had taken on so much that it was no longer fun.

As we talked it became clear that there were some boundary issues. She looked carefully at the things that she could relinquish or delegate to others, including to her husband. She had taken on more than her share just because she could "do it best." On close inspection though, there were many parts of her work that others could be trained to do. Other things she wanted to keep, even if they were tough, because she felt she really could do them well and they were satisfying to her. She learned to set specific hours for herself, to let some things go until the next day if they weren't completed, and to set her schedule so that priorities were always tended to first. In no time she looked forward to going to work in the morning—and to putting her work aside at the day's end and going home on time.

Our right job in life is always something that we enjoy. Sometimes we need to change jobs, but other times we just need to change our perspective—and find ways to simplify.

Everything has challenges and usually includes some degree of stress; but when we're in our right place, we can find the balance. If we're doing too much, we're doing more than our share. If we're not doing enough, we're not doing our share. If we're not happy, there are options: go back to school; simplify your living arrangements and work at something that is more satisfying even if it pays less. Take time to discover what fires up your enthusiasm—what are the things that you really love to do? Changes don't have to happen overnight, but if your life is tied up, start loosening the knots.

$\approx$ **29** $\approx$

Step Nine:
Establish Personal Integrity

*Integrity includes but goes beyond honesty. Honesty is telling
the truth—in other words, conforming our words to reality.
Integrity is conforming reality to our words—in other words,
keeping promises and fulfilling expectations.*

STEPHEN R. COVEY

In order to be at peace with ourselves, we need to maintain personal integrity. We live at a challenging time. The laws of personal integrity are so routinely bent all around us that many have lost sight of what it means to live with integrity—even with regard to ourselves. In that sense, cancer or any other difficulty that comes along offers an opportunity or reminder to step back and take a deeper look into life and the role we are playing. How well do we really know and trust ourselves?

There are many ways that we violate our integrity with little or no awareness of doing so. Personal integrity means many things about the ways we treat ourselves and others: being honest, telling the truth, keeping our word. Of course, being honest doesn't mean blurting out hurtful assessments or judgments of someone else's taste, for example, or insulting someone because "it's the truth." And keeping our word doesn't mean that if circumstances change we can't renegotiate something. I always remember Peace Pilgrim's lesson about applying the spirit, not the letter of the law; this involves using good discernment.

Living with integrity means that we know ourselves well and can trust ourselves to do the right thing. If we make a mistake, we don't make excuses. We learn from it without beating ourselves up emotionally and do what we can to set things right.

It is so easy to establish habits of broken carelessness in our personal integrity that we can't trust ourselves; and when we can't trust ourselves, we don't trust others. As a result we live in doubt and fear. The best way to establish a sense of trust in life and safety in relationships is to practice personal integrity. It doesn't matter what someone else is doing. What matters is how we choose to live our own lives.

The exploration of this important principle and the violation of integrity is being demonstrated on every level of private and public life. We have lied and been lied to so many times that we question what, really, is the truth. Mostly, we don't know. Most of us, to some degree, have bought into the idea that principles can be compromised under certain circumstances or conditions. We give lip service to accepted virtues, but we rationalize why they don't count in a particular situation.

They always count. In the long run, when we act without truth and integrity, we cheat ourselves. We can look to the collective view for perspective. The world is not at peace. Nations are warring against nations. Hearts are hardened. People are not speaking the truth.

The outer situation is merely a reflection of the inner situation. Peace starts within individual human hearts. Forgiveness and goodwill start within individual human minds. Integrity starts with the thoughts, words, and actions of individuals. Whatever we want—truth, justice, peace, compassion, wisdom—we all need to become. The time to start is now. Today is the day.

Peace Pilgrim noted that there are certain laws we all have to live by if we wish to find peace within or without. "So I got busy on a very interesting project. This was to live all the good things I believed in. I did not confuse myself by trying to take them all at once, but rather, if I was doing something that I knew I shouldn't be doing, I stopped doing it. And I made a quick relinquishment. That's the easy way. Tapering off is long and hard. And if I was not doing something that I knew I should be doing, I got busy on that. It took the living quite a while to catch up to the believing, but of course it can."

30

Step Ten:
Embrace Intuition

When you approach intuitive methods with respect, you become open to hearing from your interior channels.

CAROLINE MYSS

Intuition is not a gift that some people have and others don't. It is a built-in system that we all have; but as muscles atrophy from lack of use, it simply stops working if we don't pay attention. Intuition is that first gut feeling we have about something. It is a connection to an inner wisdom that comes with clarity and knowing.

There is no confusion about it. Intuition doesn't come from the ego. It can be distinguished from a reaction of fear or compulsion in that it is not based on emotion and it is always in sync with the highest spiritual principles. If, however, we allow the rational mind to jump in and negate the intuition with its logic and beliefs before we act on it, the power of this infallible source of personal wisdom goes unrecognized and the intuitive signals slip beneath the surface of our conscious awareness.

I think of intuition as part of a natural spiritual unfoldment that attunes us, if we listen to it, to a path of wisdom and compassion. The cognitive mind, on the other hand, can be like a merry-go-round where rationalizations and intellectual debates often keep the mind running in

219

circles. Of course it's important to use our intellect when appropriate, but we're not meant to run our lives by cold, hard reasoning.

The voice of intuition connects us to the individual path of our soul's journey and our spiritual reality. We've all felt it. It may be a hunch or an uncomfortable feeling that nudges us to do something. Too often, though, we don't trust our intuitions when they come, especially when they seem silly or irrational; or we simply don't act on them. But if we continue to tune them out, we stop being aware of them.

Mothers—and sometimes fathers—often have naturally fine-tuned intuitive senses involving their children. A mother may suddenly feel a foreboding and dash off to the baby's room to discover that her child has pulled a blanket over his face. Or she remembers that she left a bottle of aspirin open on the bathroom sink and dashes in just as her toddler is reaching for it.

On the other side children often have very keen perceptions, especially where their parents are concerned. When my daughter was four years old, I sat writing a letter in the bathroom while she played in the tub, when she suddenly laughed. "What's so funny?" I asked. "You don't make a hundred dollars a week," she giggled, relating back to me the words I was in the process of writing.

Cindy has maintained her intuitive awareness as an adult. One night I had a very unusual and uncomfortable dream from which I could not rouse myself. In my mind I started crying out to my daughter, asking her to call so the phone would wake me up. She didn't call. Eventually I came out of the dream and went back to a more restful sleep. At six-thirty the next morning she called and asked with great concern, "Are you all right?" I could hardly believe she had picked up on my dream summons. "I woke up at two," she continued, "and wanted so much to call you. I felt you were in trouble, but Randy said, 'Don't be silly. You'll just wake her up.'"

The mother of a newly licensed teenage driver confided to me that, when she saw her son take a bedroll to his car, she spontaneously saw in her mind the bedroll obstructing his view as he backed up. She felt compelled to tell him to put it in the trunk, but he was just going around the corner to a friend's house for the night and she let it go. That night she brought up to her husband that she wanted to call the son and tell him to put the bedroll into the trunk when he came home the next day. Again, she didn't follow through. The next morning when her son backed out of his friend's driveway, he ran into a parked car. Luckily the damage was minor. Sheepishly, the mother told me she had been praying to gain more awareness of her intuition!

Intuition can also be a sense of knowing or rightness that persists in spite of logical opposition—even when the people you care about most, or persons in authority, are telling you you're making a mistake. We often think we can save other people from their poor decisions—but it is only the ego in us asserting what we would do in similar circumstances. In truth, we offer a far greater gift when we bolster others' confidence in their ability to make their own choices and find their unique path.

Intuition is an infallible guide that never leads us astray because it originates with the higher self. With practice we can learn to both recognize and build confidence in our intuitive perceptions. Quiet reflection, journaling, and meditation are ideal practices to begin to recognize and strengthen this special awareness.

31

Step Eleven:
Love Yourself

*As a human being related to all living beings, we must
be first related to ourselves. We cannot understand, love,
and welcome others without first knowing and loving ourselves.*

JEAN KLEIN

It sounds simple enough to love ourselves, but all too often we become so wrapped up in feelings of guilt or low self-esteem that it isn't easy to do. I can certainly see, in retrospect, how far down my self-esteem had slipped when my body succumbed to cancer. In order to come to a place of inner healing, I had to review all of the things I was disappointed in about myself. Only then could I accept myself and offer myself the same respect that I was able to give to others.

What I have found in my counseling work is that most of us carry around an inner voice that is often called the critical parent. It might say things like, "Why bother? You'll never be able to do that!" Considering this, most of us could benefit from reparenting ourselves—that is, consciously directing our inner dialogue to be that of an encouraging parent: "You've always been creative. You can do anything you set your mind to."

An example that comes to my mind is a woman named Linda, who saw me for some time. From radiation treatment she had developed scars in her stomach that made it difficult for her to digest food, and her belly was bloated and uncomfortable. Her legs were swollen from her pelvis down because of blocked lymph nodes, so she had to use a walker to get around. She had done a tremendous amount of healing work around the issues in her life and, as she lay on her sofa talking to me softly, Linda said, "You know, there is only one kink in my existence right now, and that is my relationship with my cat." This was a remarkable statement in itself, considering her physical condition.

She told me she felt bad because the cat, a very large male, so wanted to be with her, but she was always pushing him off the bed or the couch because his weight hurt her. "I start to feel all this explosive energy and I blast poor Arnold with it. Then I feel terrible afterwards."

Linda went on to say that she often felt frustrated by all the little things that had become so difficult, but she would hold the feelings in; then when Arnold got in her way or wanted to lean on her, she would let her frustration burst loose. "Arnold is so accepting and he loves me so unconditionally that he still comes back and wants to be with me."

We talked about the nature of unconditionally loving relationships and how even the cat, in some part of its being, recognized that the love between them was undisturbed by her condition or outbursts. Linda loved his soothing presence and resonating purr. If he was to stay in her environment, he needed firm but loving discipline in being taught that he couldn't lie on her like he used to or get in the way of her walker. He also needed her love and soothing voice. "I know that it's my attitude toward myself that needs to change," Linda reflected. "And then I just know that Arnold won't be so needy."

I suspected that Linda had a tough critical parent inside. I asked her to close her eyes and imagine herself as a little girl in the same condition as she was in now, weak and unable to get around very well. I asked her to imagine that Arnold was getting in the little girl's way and to see her explode in the same way that Linda did as an adult. Then I asked her adult self to say something to the little girl who was having such a hard time and who had just screamed at the cat. "You shouldn't be so mean to the cat!" her critical adult scolded.

I knew that Linda was close to her grown daughter. I asked her to imagine that her daughter was a little girl with this condition. "She's so weak, and her stomach is swollen and uncomfortable, and Arnold is getting in her way. See her in your mind's eye and watch as she explodes at Arnold. What do you want to say to her?"

In a very loving voice Linda said, "I'm so sorry that you're having such a difficult time. I understand how hard it is for you, and I wish there was something I could do to help you." I asked her to make an internal switch and imagine that she was the daughter, feeling what it was like to receive that kind of understanding and acceptance. The tears rolled down Linda's cheeks. "It feels so good that someone cares about me and knows how hard it is for me."

Again, I asked her to imagine herself as a little girl and go through the visualization of screaming at Arnold. This time she gave herself the love and support she had needed all along. "It feels so good to know I can have an inner parent who loves me just the way I am and who understands what I feel." It was a powerful demonstration of the need for self-love. It was beautiful to see Linda's ability to receive it when it was presented in a way that she could really grasp.

An interesting thing about learning to give ourselves unconditional love is that it creates an opening that lets love from others in more fully. The next time I saw Linda her physical body had greatly deteriorated, but what was most striking was the radiance shining from her face and eyes. She glowed as she spoke about the special moments she was experiencing with loved ones and friends. It was apparent that she had found self-acceptance, and the peace she'd made with herself had spread to her relationships with others. The energy she was emanating was like a blessing that reached out and drew others into a very special intimacy.

The last time I saw Linda, I held her hand as she told me about a dream she'd had the night before. "I was having a very difficult night with a lot of discomfort. Then I drifted into the most wonderful dream. I never felt more free or more well. I was able to move so effortlessly. But I knew my body wasn't cured."

Dreams have been called the language of the subconscious, and Linda seemed to understand the message here. Her face was accepting and radiant. Before I could say anything she said, "I know I'm dying, but what I want to focus on is life."

As I looked at Linda, who was suffering from the same type of cancer that I had once had, I remembered my determination to learn and to teach how to die well. Now here was Linda, demonstrating the peace and joyfulness I had wanted to express if I went in this direction. "You've become my teacher," I told her, and her appreciative gaze blessed me. She left her body a week later, surrounded by people she loved.

32

Step Twelve: Do All You Can and Release the Rest

*God grant me the serenity to accept the things I cannot
change, the courage to change the things I can,
and the wisdom to know the difference.*

SERENITY PRAYER

One of the biggest stressors we put on ourselves is trying to control situations that are out of our hands. We strain with all of our might to push the immovable mountain out of our path instead of putting our energy into what we are able to do in a given situation. A life-threatening illness or catastrophic event can be such a mountain. We can drain our energy trying to get it out of our way, or we can forge a path around the mountain or perhaps climb the heights where we may find an extraordinary view of life from a new perspective.

Whenever a difficulty or problem confronts us, we can break it down into components—the parts that we can do something about, and those that we can release. To begin, we can release the things that just are—the isness of the situation. What is, simply is. We are a certain age, a certain sex. We have a particular condition or circumstance.

We can't change the past, and we don't know what will come next. Of course every thought and every action on our part influences the future, but the final outcome is out of sight. In focusing on the past or future, we are spending precious energy—and that expenditure will have an effect on the outcome. We can let both go and free our energy for the things we can see and respond to in the present. The present is always our point of power.

We can also let go of any aspects of a problem that are brought in by other people. It may be that loved ones or authority figures have a different opinion or expectation of what it is that we need or don't need to be or do. Or maybe we have an idea that certain people need to change in some way or do something that we think they should do. We lose our power and personal integrity when we live our lives to please others or attempt to change others to please ourselves. I'm not referring to the compromises that are required to create good relationships. I'm referring to the decisions and choices we need to make to be true to ourselves and to the fact we need to allow others that same freedom.

Once we are able to release the "isness" of the circumstances we are facing, and the parts of the problem that are brought in by other people, already the problem or situation has become smaller. We have eliminated the things that are out of our control, and all that remains are the things we can do something about.

On the physical side, we can look at our lifestyle. What are our habits with regard to diet, exercise, rest, and so on? "I can't quit smoking," a young client stated matter-of-factly. "This is who I am." It is possible to relate so deeply to our addictions or unhealthy habits that they become like a relationship in which we have lost our boundaries—and our balance. Illness can push us into making important changes that we haven't chosen voluntarily. When I thought I just needed to live long enough to tie up a few loose ends, I focused on how best to support my physical body during that time.

The specifics of physical self-care are unique for every individual, though all bodies need appropriate nutrition, exercise, sunshine, rest, and fresh air. These basics are crucial when our immune systems are overloaded with illness or stress.

If we pay attention, our bodies can guide us. Someone getting plenty of sleep at night, for example, but still feeling tired during the day may need to take naps. At one point during my healing process, I was sleeping as much as sixteen hours in a twenty-four hour period. In this fast-paced age when so many of us have conditioned ourselves to constant productivity, this can present a real challenge—and bring a real breakthrough. Sleep is a time when we process the many lessons we're working on in life; tiredness may be a message from our inner guidance system that we need time to withdraw from the busyness outside and pay attention to messages coming from the inside.

Figure out what time of day you experience your peak energy and schedule in some form or exercise that you can enjoy. Start slowly and build your strength. No matter where you're starting from, you can do something, and then you can add a little more. Get plenty of sunshine, preferably before 10 A.M. or after 2 P.M. to avoid the more damaging rays. Breathe deeply, one of the simplest and most beneficial things we can do for ourselves.

Getting appropriate nutrition is a very powerful way to support our bodies and our physical healing process. There are all kinds of books and resources for guidance in this area. General suggestions include increasing dietary fiber, fresh fruits, fresh vegetables, and whole grains, all organically grown when possible. Avoid smoking, alcohol, and smoked, salted, pickled, or barbecued foods. Consult a nutritionist for diet and supplementation recommendations specifically suited to your individual needs.

On the psychological side, what we bring into a situation includes our fears, our anger, our past experiences, and our hopes and expectations. We may initially feel powerless when confronting these things, but all we need to do is face them—as the first step toward releasing or resolving them.

What do we fear? Dying? Feeling pain? Having financial difficulties? Losing a relationship? Once again, the first step is to separate out the things that are out of our control and release them: the time of our death; the reality of pain; the amount of our income and the money owed in the present moment; another person's choice to be or not to be in relationship with us. Next, what are the things that we can and are willing to do in regard to these fears? This is where we can place our energy.

One way to overcome a fear is to get acquainted with it. If we fear dying, we can read books on the subject, talk to hospice workers, tune in to that great pool of inner wisdom through meditation, and so on. If we fear pain, we can experiment with ways to ease the sensation of discomfort. Exercises could include relaxation, meditation or self-hypnosis, reflexology, medication, or various diversions such as conversations with family and friends, funny videos, or inspirational books and music. If our fears concern money, we can search out resources around us if they are available in our greater families; we can do research to find local or state programs that are set up to help people out in times of need; or we can find some creative way to refinance our bills or simplify our lifestyle. If our fear has to do with relationships, we can take responsibility for conveying what it is that we want to contribute and what it is that we would like from our partners. Ultimately, a relationship needs to be entered into by two people, and if one person is unwilling, the other needs to find a way to let go and move on.

Other things we may need to face are anger, past experiences, and hopes and expectations. We can't change the events that led to anger (an emotion that often covers up hurt), and we can't change experiences from the past, but we can make amends or find closure, either by ourselves or through communication with others when that is appropriate. When I was going through my healing process, most of the work I did with my emotions or unresolved past experiences happened through dialoguing in my journal. When it comes to hopes and expectations, we can take steps toward the things we would like to see happen and leave the outcome in higher hands.

These are only a few ideas. There is no end to our creative potential to solve the problems that are set before us. If we do not separate out the things that are out of our control and release them, a problem can seem overwhelming. I mentioned earlier how my mother in her seventies went through major surgery so beautifully, but afterward she was hit by a series of setbacks. An intestinal infection left her drained, and severe side effects from a powerful antibiotic further depleted her. When a cold moved into her head and chest it was somewhat like the straw that broke the camel's back. She felt weak, vulnerable, depressed, and powerless over her increasingly failing sense of well being.

I asked Mom what she could do right now to help herself through this difficult situation. "I can breathe," she started. That might seem obvious, but in her case breathing exercises kept her lungs strong so that fluid wouldn't accumulate. "I can eat." Again, obvious, but her condition had left her with little appetite, and she was already very petite, with no reserves in body fat. "I can walk." It was winter and cold outside, so to maintain what strength she could, she walked several rounds through her house each day. "And I can have my quiet time every morning to keep in touch with my inner guidance." She had come up with four very simple and important steps that gave her a sense of control.

When we next spoke, my mother's cough had become so disruptive that she hadn't been able to sleep for a couple of nights, adding to her exhaustion and feeling of helplessness. But she was keeping up with the four things she could do to help herself through this period. During a quiet meditation in the middle of the night when she couldn't sleep, she asked her inner guidance to give her some insight on anything further she could do for herself. The idea came to her of breathing in steam, so she set up a steamer. The warm vapors relieved her coughing almost immediately, and she was able to get the rest she needed.

But still she got worse as her cold turned into bronchitis. "Using a steamer was the best thing you could have done for yourself," her surgeon told her as he examined her two days later, confirming her intuition and giving her the encouragement she needed. Her recovery was further hampered as she went through yet another bout with the intestinal infection. But throughout she kept herself focused on what she could do to keep herself inspired and motivated. She started keeping a gratitude journal and used this special time to learn to play the piano.

My mother's strength was slow to return. In a relaxation session with me one day, I asked her to scan her body and report to me what she was feeling inside. Her whole body felt clear and well except the area around her abdomen. I asked her to imagine that she could put her abdomen in front of her and speak to it. What did she want to say?

She expressed her concern about its well-being and her frustration that she didn't know what else to do. Then I asked her to imagine that she could become her abdomen and respond. It still surprises me to hear the clarity and simple wisdom that can come when we give voice to different parts of the body. "You need to trust me," she said with authority, "and have confidence in the natural order of things. Healing takes time."

Three and a half months after her surgery Mom went in for a check-up with her primary doctor. She was better in every way, except that her bowel function had remained loose since the infections. Her doctor said, "That shouldn't still be happening. And I'm concerned that you haven't gained more weight." She ordered several tests.

My mother came home feeling depressed. After talking it over she realized that, whenever she went to her primary doctor, despite her doctor's good intentions, she came home feeling bad. She decided to pick up the test results when they came back and take them to her surgeon, who was very positive and supportive.

When the surgeon went over them with her, he assured her that she was doing fine. She mentioned her weight. He said, "Alice, you're a small woman. I'm not worried about your weight. You'll get it back slowly." Feeling more confident she said, "You know, I'm ready to just accept that loose bowels may be a permanent condition, but I'm getting my strength back and feel I can live a normal life again."

Acceptance of what is can be a powerful catalyst for change. Within a week her body functions returned to normal. Once she had turned that corner, her strength came back in leaps and bounds. A year after her surgery Mom is hiking up and down the hills of her mountain community, grateful daily for her health and appreciation of life.

It can be an uphill struggle to keep our perspective optimistic and our spirits lifted during such difficult times. It requires letting go of all the things that are out of our hands and breaking down what is left—what we can work to change—into manageable steps. There is a solution to every difficulty we encounter, a way through or around or over the top of the mountain. We have incredible potential and creativity within us just waiting to be tapped. When we get too caught up in the events unfolding around us, we sometimes see only a narrow view and lose the bigger perspective. When circumstances around us force change, we can let go of the reins and trust a higher guiding force in our lives—this is also called faith—and know that we are in our right place.

What I continue to observe in myself and others is that when we face the challenges that come to us head-on without trying to run or hide from them, we have tremendous opportunities for learning and growth. As we test our boundaries—finding the courage to do our best in life no matter what comes—we continually expand our potential. Life is like a jigsaw puzzle with the central pieces coming together first and the edges constantly growing. When we're blindsided we continue to rework the central pieces, creating the same picture over and over.

If we want to grow we have to be willing to expand our boundaries. The same principle is at work in miracles and healing. If we want to experience them, we have to be willing to step beyond our usual boundaries and open up to the possibilities.

Epilogue

Heal Ourselves, Heal the World

*The world will change when each individual makes the attempt
to counter (his or her) negative thoughts and emotions and
when we practice compassion for its inhabitants . . .*

DALAI LAMA

We are, each one of us, much more powerful than we realize. Every thought we think, every action we take, adds to the collective pool of harmony or chaos. We are constantly influencing that pool and most often we do so without any idea of the power we wield, or of how we are simultaneously influencing the balance of our own well-being—our bodies, minds and spirits.

The process of healing ourselves is a noble undertaking that enriches the world around us. We have the ability to tap into incredible inner potential and strength that in any situation can help us rise above our fears and move from victim (a recipient of circumstances) to empowered (a state of moving into meaningful action). The difficulties that we see in the world around us—the violence, the inhumanity, the greed—is a reflection of the collective inner situation. As we begin to heal on a personal level, as we take responsibility for our thoughts and actions, as we practice forgiveness and compassion, we are adding to the healing of the world.

233

All human beings have an inner drive to seek meaning and purpose. Let go of barriers for a moment and allow for the possibility that you, yourself, are here to serve a higher calling, to fulfill some unique purpose. You are being called to add to the balance and harmony of life around you. Imagine for a moment that you are suddenly aware of the time you have in this life to create that meaning and purpose. Yes, there is time to make a difference. It's exhilarating to recognize the opportunity that has just fallen into your hands. Now what to do with it?

There is so much that can be done to make a difference in life. The smallest gesture of reaching out can make a big impact on the recipient and in return have a healing effect on our own immune systems and sense of well-being. The universe is designed to reward compassion and good deeds that are offered without strings or desire of something in return. Give freely, the universe beckons, and you cannot help but receive the real treasures in return—health, happiness, and inner peace.

Very often we hold up barriers to our personal healing by being unaware of the patterns of our thinking or the destructiveness of our attitudes. We may be taking responsibility for our actions, but our feelings may be harboring resentment toward the actions of others. Our actions and feelings are the only ones we can ever be responsible for, and that is where healing and freedom lie.

A woman named Mary came to see me about an issue of not feeling worthy. She had every reason to feel successful but she didn't. She was an only child who had been brought up in a home filled with criticism. No matter what she did, in her mother's eyes, it wasn't good enough. Now, as she was reaching new levels of success, her mother had started ignoring her birthdays. She didn't even send cards. Mary's fortieth birthday had just passed without a word from her mother and it was bringing up resentment and feelings of not deserving the successes she had built.

I brought to her attention that her mother was getting older and probably wasn't going to change. What Mary could focus on was how she wanted to respond. She was no longer an abused child. She had done tremendous healing in most areas of her life and had become a compassionate and in-charge adult. I asked her to see herself in the empowered role she had created for herself, both in her private and public life. She had come so far and she could see that her mother had not come very far at all from the wounds of her own childhood. From this perspective Mary felt genuine compassion for her mother, who was still very much a wounded soul. Still, Mary didn't know how to respond to this situation.

As we brainstormed, I asked her if she could imagine calling her mother and saying something she could truthfully mean, like, "I just want to thank you for bringing me into this world forty years ago. I have a wonderful life and I'm very grateful for that." The impact of those words touched her deeply and brought tears to her eyes. She immediately made a decision to make that call. A change in perception and awareness can be so healing. Mary's feelings of resentment and not being worthy completely dissipated when she changed her feelings to compassion and took action.

A simple restructuring of awareness can turn life into an adventure in healing. We are all capable of being healers. We are helping to heal others when we listen with attentiveness and respect and without judgment. We don't have to find extra time to add meaning and purpose to our lives, we only have to change our focus and intention.

Imagine again that you are suddenly aware of the shortness of life and you realize you have an opportunity to make a difference. Go through the day with this awareness. On your way to the office you pass an accident and send a silent blessing to those involved. At the office one of your co-workers is particularly grumpy. Instead of being short with her you extend your kindness, repeatedly if necessary, and notice the eventual outcome. Most likely you will experience a calming in the environment. At the very least you will experience a calming inside of yourself. Continue through your day with this awareness, being a silent observer even while you are interacting. At home instead of snapping at the kids to do their homework, find some good thing they've done and comment on it. Do the same with a spouse or significant other. At the end of the day notice how you feel when you get into bed. Use the last moment of your awareness before drifting into sleep to send a thought of love or support to someone who needs it.

It may be surprising to notice the dramatic shifts that begin to happen as our lives take on meaning and purpose. As we keep the channels of our awareness open and make these small steps more and more inspiration comes. And as we act on those inspirations our healing deepens and our lives blossom.

It is never too late to heal and to grow. Even at the moment of death an active will of compassion and forgiveness can break through the hardest crust of bitterness. The light that radiates through blesses all who come in contact with the one who has found that strength. I have witnessed such a scene. The blessings are like seeds of grace that go forth and multiply.

The intensity reserved for moments of knowing that death is imminently near can be terrifying and immobilizing; it can also be utterly transforming and freeing. How we deal with life is much the same. We have the potential for transformation at our fingertips all the time. It can be found in moments of inspiration or in moments of crisis. It can be short-lived or enduring. The choice is always ours. It comes from the attitudes we develop, many of which are unconscious. In approaching healing in any area of our lives—our physical bodies, our mental health, our relationships, our finances—we can focus on expanding our awareness of where our thoughts are taking us, whether our beliefs are limiting or freeing and whether our attitudes are on the positive or negative side. Awareness is something we can continually bring ourselves back to.

Time is a wonderful and distorting kind of thing. It seems endless on the one hand, and there is never enough on the other. The truth is that an individual life, whether it ends at age ninety-eight or forty-eight, is short. Every moment is an opportunity to rise to the challenge of developing and offering our unique gifts. Every moment is a golden opportunity to express compassion and caring. In fact this moment right now is the moment we have to make amends, to tie up loose ends, to forgive, to heal, and to free ourselves to be fully alive.

Appendix

Summary of Steps in the Healing Process

STEP 1: TAKE CHARGE

It isn't possible to make good, conscious decisions in the midst of confusion and shock. Slow down and don't be rushed. Listen to your inner voice. Weigh the options and make decisions and choices based on what you feel is right for you. We stay far more empowered when we take charge and make decisions we feel good about.

STEP 2: DEVELOP AN EMPOWERED ATTITUDE

An empowered attitude is always in sync with inner guidance or a sense of rightness about something. Developing an empowered attitude requires a conscious effort to change any habits we have adopted that make us feel weak, overwhelmed or powerless. An empowered attitude is one that knows that whatever the circumstances, you can and will find a way to keep or regain a sense of centeredness and strength within yourself.

STEP 3: CREATE A HEALING ENVIRONMENT

A healing environment is the foundation upon which we can live our lives more fully present and alive. The place to start constructing that environment is from within. We begin to create order out of chaos by first building an inner sanctuary where we can retreat at any time to reconnect with our centeredness and grounding. A healing environment is also something we can create externally by consciously transforming the space around us that we have control over—our offices and home environments—to be places that inspire us, lift our spirits, and connect us with our hearts.

Step 4: Practice Forgiveness

Forgiveness is often one of the hardest things to practice, but it is a powerful means of personal transformation. When we forgive we are saying, in essence, that we are no longer willing to carry around pain in response to someone else's actions. Forgiveness is a core life lesson. It means cutting the cord of resentment and trusting God or spirit to bring that person the experiences he or she needs to heal.

Step 5: Explore Attitudes and Beliefs

Beliefs and attitudes can become so embedded in our subconscious minds that it's easy to lose sight of them. We can even hold conflicting beliefs without being aware of it. The words we use to communicate are symbols of our internal beliefs and as we pay attention to the words we use (and the thoughts we think) we may discover attitudes and beliefs within ourselves that don't support our healing.

Step 6: Transform Negative Feelings/Heal and Release the Past

Paying attention to how we spend our energy can provide major clues in the process of healing. When we hold onto bitterness or anger or fear toward another it is ourselves, not the object of our focus that is hurt. Holding onto negative feelings is simply an exhausting expenditure of energy that can lead to emotional and physical bankruptcy. To really heal we need to open up to the transforming power of compassion and forgiveness, both toward ourselves and others.

STEP 7: BUILD A SUPPORT SYSTEM

It's common to feel isolated when facing a life-threatening or debilitating condition, even when surrounded by loved ones. We need and can appreciate the support from family and friends, but we also need support from more neutral sources—who can hear what we're feeling without being hurt or shocked, or who have had similar experiences. A supportive counselor can be invaluable, as can a support group with empowering guidelines.

STEP 8: SIMPLIFY LIFE

Our lives are often so cluttered and busy that we find ourselves racing to keep up. What we lose are the simple basics of life that provide the balance we desperately need: walks in nature, unhurried time with our loved ones, precious quiet time alone for meditation or reading or just being mindfully grateful for the many gifts around us. Changes don't have to happen overnight but if your life is tied up, start loosening the knots.

STEP 9: ESTABLISH PERSONAL INTEGRITY

In order to be at peace with ourselves we need to live from a place of personal integrity. Living with integrity means that we know ourselves well and can trust ourselves to do the right thing. If we can't trust ourselves we don't trust others. The best way to establish a sense of trust in life and safety in relationships is to practice personal integrity. It doesn't matter what someone else is doing. What matters is how we choose to live our own lives.

STEP 10: EMBRACE INTUITION

Intuition is not a gift that some people have and others don't. It's a built in system that we all have; but as muscles that atrophy from lack of use, it simply becomes weak if we don't pay attention. We've all felt it. It might be a hunch or an uncomfortable feeling that nudges us to do something. Too often, though, we don't trust our intuitions when they come, especially when they seem silly or irrational. Too often, we simply don't act on them. But if we continue to tune them out, we stop being aware of them.

STEP 11: LOVE YOURSELF

It sounds simple enough to love ourselves, but all too often we become so wrapped up in feelings of guilt or low self-esteem that it isn't easy to do. Most of us carry around an inner critical voice that is often called the critical parent. Considering this, most of us could benefit from consciously directing our inner dialogue to be that of an encouraging parent. An interesting thing about learning to give ourselves unconditional love is that it creates an opening that lets others in more fully.

STEP 12: DO ALL YOU CAN AND RELEASE THE REST

One of the biggest stressors we put on ourselves is trying to control situations or outcomes that are out of our hands. Whenever a difficulty or problem confronts us, we can break it down into components: the parts we can do something about, and those that we can release. There is a solution to every difficulty we encounter, a way through or around or over the top of the mountain. We have incredible potential and creativity within us, just waiting to be tapped.

Bibliography

Churchill, Randal, *Become the Dream*, Transforming Press, 1997. P.O. Box 9369, Santa Rosa, CA 95405 Phone: 209-962-6403 Website: www.hypnoschool.com.

Dyer, Dr. Wayne, *You'll See It When You Believe it*, William Morrow and Co., Inc., 1989. Dr. Dyer is also the author of Your Erroneous Zones and Wisdom of the Ages: 60 Days to Enlightenment.

Jampolsky, Gerald G., *Love Is Letting Go of Fear*, Celestial Arts, 1988.

Jampolsky, Gerald G., *Forgiveness: The Greatest Healer of All*, 1999.

Myss, Caroline, Ph.D., *Anatomy of the Spirit*, Harmony Books, 1996.

Myss, Caroling, Ph.D., *Why People Don't Heal and How They Can*, Harmony Books, November, 1997.

Myss, Caroline, Ph.D., *Sacred Contracts: Awakening Your Divine Potential*, Harmony Books, 2001.

Northrup, Christiane, M.D., *Women's Bodies, Women's Wisdom*, Bantam Books, 1994.

Pearce, Joseph Chilton, *Evolution's End: Claiming the Potential of Our Intelligence*, Harper, 1993.

Pearce, Joseph Chilton, *Magical Child*, Plume, 1992.

Pearce, Joseph Chilton, *The Biology of Transcendence: A Blueprint of the Human Spirit*, Inner Traditions Intl. Ltd., 2002.

Pilgrim, Peace, *Peace Pilgrim, Her Life and Work in her Own Words*, Friends of Peace Pilgrim, 1982. The book and a listing of other offerings can be obtained from Friends of Peace Pilgrim, 43480 Cedar Ave., Somerset, CA 95684.

Pilgrim, Peace, *Peace Pilgrim's Wisdom, Daily Meditations*, Blue Dove/Ocean Tree, 1996. Compiled and edited by Cheryl Canfield, Ocean Tree Books, P.O. Box 1295, Santa Fe, NM, 87504, phone: 505-983-1412 or Blue Dove Press, P.O. Box 261611, San Diego, CA 92196.

Williamson, Marianne, *Return to Love: Reflections on the Principles of a Course in Miracles*. HarperCollins, 1996. Williamson is also the author of *A Woman's Worth* and *Illuminata: A Return to Prayer.*

Zubko, Andy, *Treasury of Spiritual Wisdom*, Blue Dove Press, 1996. Blue Dove Press, P.O. Box 261611, San Diego, CA 92196.

Books of Related Interest

HEALING WITHOUT FEAR
How to Overcome Your Fear of Doctors, Hospitals, and the Health
Care System and Find Your Way to True Healing
by Laurel Ann Reinhardt, Ph.D.

**EMOTIONAL HEALING THROUGH MINDFULNESS
MEDITATION**
Stories and Meditations for Women Seeking Wholeness
by Barbara Miller Fishman, Ph.D.

FIGHT CANCER WITH VITAMINS AND SUPPLEMENTS
A Guide to Prevention and Treatment
by Kedar N. Prasad, Ph.D., and K. Che Prasad, M.D.

WHY IS CANCER KILLING OUR PETS?
How You Can Protect and Treat Your Animal Companion
by Deborah Straw

ACCEPTING YOUR POWER TO HEAL
The Personal Practice of Therapeutic Touch
by Dolores Krieger, Ph.D., R.N.

OXYGEN HEALING THERAPIES
For Optimum Health and Vitality
by Nathaniel Altman

HILDEGARD OF BINGEN'S SPIRITUAL REMEDIES
by Dr. Wighard Strehlow

WHEN HEALING BECOMES A CRIME
The Amazing Story of the Hoxsey Cancer Clinics
and the Return of Alternative Therapies
by Kenny Ausubel

Inner Traditions • Bear & Company
P.O. Box 388
Rochester, VT 05767
1-800-246-8648
www.InnerTraditions.com

Or contact your local bookseller